Songs at Twilight

Songs at Twilight:
A Narrative Exploration of Living with a Visual Impairment
and the Effect this has on Claims to Identity

By

Susan Dale

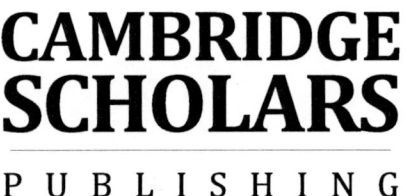

CAMBRIDGE
SCHOLARS

PUBLISHING

Songs at Twilight:
A Narrative Exploration of Living with a Visual Impairment and the Effect this has on Claims to Identity,
by Susan Dale

This book first published 2011

Cambridge Scholars Publishing

12 Back Chapman Street, Newcastle upon Tyne, NE6 2XX, UK

British Library Cataloguing in Publication Data
A catalogue record for this book is available from the British Library

ISBN (10): 1-4438-2917-X, ISBN (13): 978-1-4438-2917-5

To John,

For loving me

*in sickness, as well as in health
and enduring the writing!*

TABLE OF CONTENTS

Part 3 Enabling Practices and Transforming Identities

Acknowledgements

I want to honour and thank all of those who have given me strength and the will to continue and complete both my doctorate and this book over the last 5 years. These include:

Andy, Sarah, Dennis, Tony, Adam and Mike – Thank you. Without your support, your love and your courage this study would never have come into being.

All the contributors who so willingly have read, commented on and spoken to me about their life experiences and for allowing your comments to become part of this narrative

My academic supervisor Tim – without you saying to me, "you can write" I would have never ever started! and without your support I would have given up long ago!

John my husband, for proof reading and correcting my appalling spelling and grammar!

Becky my gorgeous daughter, for your love and for being an inspiration to your mother.

Sam and Adam for bearing with your aged mother, and keeping me computer literate!

RNIB CYMRU, for recording the audio-book and providing Master CD.

Jan Hillman my counselling supervisor, for your "super-vision" and continuing love and support.

Jane Speedy, Malcolm Reed, for your inspiring teaching and infectious love of a good story.

Mary Norowzian, for your support and encouragement; both in my work as a counsellor, and in my writing.

All my friends at RNIB and Action for Blind People who continue to offer support and encouragement.

PROLOGUE

Sue Journal June 2010
I have a certain amount of useful sight which means during the day I rarely think about what I cannot see. Because I have no night vision however the twilight hour is the time of day I remember my blindness. It is the sign that darkness will soon come and again and I will again be blind. It is a time of mourning, of lamentation, but it is also a time remembered of sitting around a campfire and singing songs and the warmth of the fire on my face where I felt drawn to others, not by vision, but by a sense of belonging, a sense of community.

A song my mother used to sing to calm my childhood fears at the onset of darkness comes into my mind:

> "Just a song at twilight, when the lights are low;
> And the flick'ring shadows softly come and go.
> Tho' the heart be weary, sad the day and long,
> Still to us at twilight comes love's old song,
> Comes love's old sweet song" (Bingham 1927)

The beginning of a story about visual impairment

"Writing this book has made me blind" says Kleege (1999:1). She does not mean that in a physical sense she lost her sight whilst writing the book, but more that she explored her own relationship with blindness and how different her view of the world is than that of the majority.

Although night time has always reminded me of my visual limitations my journey into blindness and the relationship I have with being visually impaired really only came to the fore when I took up post as senior counsellor and project co-ordinator with RNIB (Royal National Institute of the Blind) Bristol in October 2005, and worked alongside volunteer counsellors to provide an innovative counselling service for people affected by sight loss. Until then I realise I had always lived my life as a sighted person without the sight and tried with moderate success to ignore what I could not see and to fit into the expectations that being sighted was "normal" and being visually impaired was definitely "not normal".

I have always written to try to make sense of the world I live and work in and this book is born out of my attempt to make sense of how I and other people who are visually impaired live in a world that prizes sight above all other senses. It is written from the perspective of considering that our sense of self and identity is socially constructed through relationship and the stories we tell of our lives.

The story of this book starts here; firstly with my own reflections on my work for the RNIB, then expanding to a small narrative research project I undertook with two ex-counselling clients who call themselves Andy and Sarah, which led to the emergence of a narrative entitled "Knitting in the Dark" (Dale 2006) which in turn led to a doctoral research project and then the text you are now reading.

Journal November 2005

"It must be bloody terrible. I don't think that I could ever cope with it. I just couldn't go on living if it were me". This was my taxi drivers thought for the day as we crawled through traffic towards my visit to a client at home. The driver is someone I travel with regularly, and regularly transports other visually impaired colleagues and members of RNIB. I am curious (although I didn't challenge him at the time) by his implication that sight loss was a tragedy. Certainly I don't consider it a tragedy, being born with a visual impairment that leaves me with tunnel vision is just part of who I am as a person. I'm not suggesting that at times this hasn't been frustrating, especially when I am entirely dependent on public transport - but having no peripheral vision has also enabled me to focus on one thing at a time, develop seeing through hearing, listening, and intuition possibly good attributes for a counsellor! I wonder about the different stories that I am hearing about sight loss and how prominent "tragedy" and "medical" stories are, and how little is told about peoples personal experience.

Journal: December 2005

I have discovered there is so much I do not know about visual impairment, especially sight loss. Many of my clients report having "lost" their vision, and finding this a frightening isolating time; a time where there is so much grief for what is lost, at the same time as trying to learn new ways of living.

I want to understand something of what's happening to the people I'm working with. I look up various "conditions" on RNIB's website. I am struck by how calm and still the words on the page are, and how this contrast's with the person's experience. "Charles Bonnet Syndrome" is named after a Swiss philosopher who first described *this condition in 1760 when he noticed his grandfather who was blinded by cataracts describing seeing birds and buildings which were not there. (RNIB 2006:3). Tears prick the back of my eyes as I hold these words alongside the story of one of my clients (Sarah) who had thought for over 12 months that she was going mad.*

Apparently these visual hallucinations are common. If they are common, why are they not explained to people? I feel angry. Several clients have spoken of seeing things and being so afraid. Afraid they were losing their mind as well as their sight.

Journal: January 2006
There's so many things which I thought I knew about not being able to see very well that I realise I don't know at all. How do you cope if you are elderly, alone and then you lose your vision? How is it when your whole life has been reading, writing and you can no longer do these things? The hours in the day must seem so long and endless.

Often there seems to be a battle between learning new skills and the "not wanting to go on". I had a conversation with (Andy) today who is a 60 year old man with diabetic retinopathy. His rehabilitation worker referred him as he seemed to have "got on well to start with, but now was refusing to go out". "He seems really fed up" she said. Andy talked to me about how hard it is for him to keep up an act of "coping well" and although he knows he can learn new ways of doing things, he feels so angry and despairing.

"The only thing I have control over now is if I live or if I die" he says. Suicidal thoughts seem top of everyone's agenda at the moment and sometimes I feel like the little Dutch boy who puts his finger in the dyke only to find more and more holes appearing.

Journal: February 2006
Today I feel stressed and it feels much more appealing to go with the social model of disability and see people's sight problems as "going away" if we as a society promote more accessible services and communications. If we can give people the tools to live their lives by way of aids for living… I realise as I write this that although I do strongly agree that society needs to enable rather than disable others this is my feeble attempt to try to keep feeling in control.

The day has gone pear-shaped. My taxi was late arriving to pick me up from a client's home, which meant I was late for the information day (for the newly diagnosed) my next client then arrived very distressed and talked of how he had tried to commit suicide using a carving knife. Hearing his pain was very hard, but I am amazed that he is still here, and is committed to "finding a way through this". His talking was like an eruption which I thought would never cease "nobody has ever listened before", he says. "They have been marvellous at the hospital, and tried everything but they say they can't do any more...they don't want to know that I'm not coping". I wonder about the staff at the hospitals, how do they cope with giving others bad news, they see so many patients in a day, but I also wonder about the silent suffering.

Journal: March 2006

My work sometimes seems like a drop in the ocean. As I sit here on the train I have been thinking about how I struggle between wanting to be "right in there with the client" and also working in a time sensitive way. At times I feel I am not allowing clients to tell me things that I think would be difficult to manage in a brief intervention. There are always more clients appearing on the waiting list which is a dilemma that haunts thousands of medical professionals all over the country. Do we offer this person more treatment at the expense of making this person wait? What are the priorities? Does the inevitable compromise mean nobody is getting a good service?

Identity seems a key issue, when we know ourselves as a "sighted person" who are we when we are no longer "sighted". I have read a very interesting article by Langellier (2001) which showed how the narrator transformed the effects of treatment for breast cancer (including mastectomy) with a tattoo over the scar. She moved from someone who was "treated" to someone who had transformed tragedy into a new identity. I wonder can the "eye care pathway" (jargon charting the patients through diagnosis, treatment and registration) make room for this kind of transformation?

Journal: April 2006

The narrative therapy practice of using therapeutic documents has taken a new turn today. In the past I often asked people to write journals and/or written to them between sessions, today I had suggested to a client that she keep an audio journal and she played part of it to me today. It was fascinating how by listening to the original story (which she had recorded) she was then changing and enriching the story as she talked to me. She was reconnecting with her skills as a writer (she had in the past written both poetry and short stories). I asked her "does this 'telling on tape' change how 'depression' holds on to you?" She replied "it can't touch me when I write, and I can write even though it is in a different way". She had called her original story "when the angels came" and now she had found a preferred alternative story of "knitting in the dark" but that knitting in the dark was ok. It was a bit "messy" and "complicated" but that the "multi-coloured garment" produced was worth it.

I've been thinking about my sight too. I realise that I have been effectively living as a "sighted person" without the sight. For the first time ever I asked the university to provide me with documents in large print. Their response was positive. I felt like crying.

Journal: May 2006

Frustration, anger, humiliation those are my thoughts for the day. I stood with fellow students at the crossing on Park Street in Bristol. The lights weren't working. The rest of the group crossed leaving me stranded on the other side of the street. They wait talking amongst themselves as taking a deep breath I plunge into the traffic. A driver hurls an obscenity through the window. "Sorry", says my friend "I forgot", and charges forward through the throng of students. I say nothing, but feel everything. The fault however lies with me. My white stick, as normal, lies folded neatly, zipped in my bag.

A funny(?) incident happened today. I came out of my client's home to find no taxi, so waited patiently by the side of the road. Ten minutes later a car drew up and I jumped in. Fortunately it was the taxi. He was horrified. "You shouldn't wait by the side of the road here" he said "This is the street where ladies of uncertain reputations pick up their clients". A salutary lesson—check the taxi credentials before jumping in, and be careful where you wait! One of the many challenges for those with poor eyesight!

Journal: June 2006

I have met today with two ex-clients Andy who I saw for 8 counselling sessions at the RNIB centre, and Sarah who I met with for 12 counselling sessions in her home. They want to tell their stories so that others might understand. I feel excited yet fearful. I don't want to let them down. We have decided that the title for the research project will be "Knitting in the Dark".

"Knitting in the Dark: an exploration of the experience of living with a visual impairment"[1] was my first tentative step on the doctoral programme which I had enrolled and was intended to augment the statistical data collected as part of the counselling project using CORE-OM which is a benchmarked research tool developed for psychotherapeutic practices, (Barkham et al. 2006). I had hoped that the stories would give sighted others some idea about what living with a visual impairment might be like and to act as a pilot project for a possible doctoral thesis.

I was taken aback by the wealth of responses I received, not just from sighted eye care professionals, but from other people who lived with a visual impairment. People emailed, telephoned, sent me audio-tapes of their own experience, and stopped me in the corridors of RNIB offices to talk with me about my writing. There was an air of excitement and enthusiasm about the stories that I had not expected. My doctoral project was born. I then worked with Adam, Mike, Dennis and Tony and we compiled an audio narrative exploration of our experiences of living with a visual impairment and the effect this had on identity claims. This was another life changing project. We used an audio-narrative medium to challenge the taken for granted text based academic practices[2]. Once again the stories emerging from the study were listened to and read avidly by people who were visually impaired who in turn sent in their comments, reflections and their own stories.

This book is autoethnographic, and yet also collective. Not collective in the sense of distilling the many voices to one, but collective in the sense of linking the experiences of unique individuals across a common theme to provide "thick rich descriptions" of a subject matter that is so often thought of in mono-dimensional terms. It attempts to sew together in a giant tapestry the stories emerging from the pilot project "Knitting in the Dark", my doctoral thesis and also stories from the many people who responded to these projects. It hopefully gives not the "truth" about visual impairment, or narrative research, or any of us individuals (who are so much more than visually impaired) but a glimpse of the lived experience of a group of individuals who are trying to make sense of their lives living with reduced vision. It is an attempt by us to develop an opportunity for people with a visual impairment to find a voice in a world that is predominately sighted in its outlook, and to challenge sighted communities about their taken for granted attitudes about sight. These are stories not of tragedy, but of hope and resilience.

---

[1] See Dale 2006 2008a and 2008b for more details.
[2] The dissertation was submitted to the university as an audio-book with a text transcript (Dale 2009).

INTRODUCTION

The narratives you will find contained in the pages of this book will hopefully speak for themselves giving a glimpse of the lived experience of a group of people living with a visual impairment. Within this introduction I intend to give some context for the narratives with an overview of the book and the underpinning research methodology. There is also an exploration of some of the current literature relating to visual impairment research, and an introduction to the contributors.

Claims to Identity

The concept of "identity" and how we define ourselves is very complex. My own views (and practice as a counsellor and researcher) are influenced by post-structuralist understandings of how we make sense of our lives, where I see identity as constructed through relationship, and the stories we tell of our lives. As Brockmeier and Carbaugh state, "the stories we tell ourselves about ourselves and others organize our senses of who we are, who others are, and how we are related" (Brockmeier and Carbaugh 2001:10).

I am visually impaired and registered as partially sighted. One of the questions I have been grappling with recently is: If our identity is socially constructed, then how does this relate to being visually impaired? After all, as Kinash points out, "not being able to see is not socially constructed" (Kinash 2005:19), the "not seeing" is after all a physiological fact. The attitudes that society has towards blindness however are socially constructed; thus within a world where the majority are sighted, social interactions have developed to consider vision as "normal" and those of us who have different vision as abnormal. I suppose in some senses this is a democratic process, but in placing so much value on sight and in considering this constructed value as a "truth", the experience of those who are blind or partially sighted is often negated thus influencing research and how services are provided.

Literature relating to visual impairment

Literature reviews reveal that the majority of research relating to visual impairment comes from medical understandings of vision loss, with emphasis on diagnosis, treatment and rehabilitation. This has usually been undertaken by sighted "experts" speaking about people who are blind or partially sighted (Bolt 2005; Monbeck 1973; Scott 1969; Fitzgerald and Murray Parkes 1998) to name but a few. There is a growing collection of studies written about the emotional responses to sight loss (Burmedi et al. 2002; Butler 2007; Stephens 2007; Thurston 2010), and there are a number of non-academic memoirs and biographies including works by Ching (1980); Hull (1990); Kuusisto (1998); Knighton (2006; 2007) and of course the works of Helen Keller (1912; 1933). There are, however, few visually impaired researchers overtly using their personal experiences to influence research, with the exception of Kleege (1999; 2006); French and Swain (2000); Tuttle and Tuttle (2004); Krieger (2005) and Thurston (2010).

Deaf studies, and disability studies (Campbell and Oliver 1996; White 1997; Barnes and Mercer 2003; Hole 2004; Mintz 2007; French and Swain 2004; Barnes, Mercer, and Shakespeare 1999) give a different perspective, and have helped me consider how the social movement of disability has gained momentum, a movement which espouses that disability is not about physical difference, but about societal negative attitudes towards that difference. This movement has encouraged more public awareness of disability discrimination, and actively sought to change public attitudes. It has encouraged the promotion of inclusive practices within education, the workplace and social settings which has resulted in less overt discrimination and more accessible services being available for example, disabled toilets, lifts and accessible documents and signs, and workplace assistance being available to help both employers and their disabled employees. The issues of disability rights are now implemented through statute in the form of the Disability Discrimination Act 2005, and the Equality Act 2010 but despite these rights now being widely promoted, it does not always seem to have an effect on how people feel about living as "visually impaired", or their experience of discrimination. Tony (one of the contributors) said to me recently, "the Act is just a token really, people are more careful about what they say to you, but they still think the same! It only pays lip-service to my needs, and ignores completely how I feel or what I need".

Duckett and Pratt in 1999 and 2007 conducted reviews of visual impairment research and called for research practices where there was empowerment and "greater inclusion of visually impaired people" (Duckett and Pratt 2007:7) and French and Swain called for research (with people who were disabled) to be emancipatory, and that "supported people in their struggle against oppression and inequality" (French and Swain 2000:35). This book is a response to these calls and intends to give voice to those living with a visual impairment. It also hopefully opens up a space for further conversation between visually impaired and sighted communities in order to empower and give voice to those who are visually impaired, and to encourage research which does not negate their experience.

This book intentionally moves away from "expert" and "medical" opinion, or even "social theories" of disability. It uses a collaborative, narrative, methodology that enables myself and 30 contributors to explore our personal experiences of living with a visual impairment and in doing so "gives voice" to people who are blind and partially sighted. The themes contained in each chapter are those contributors felt important to share with readers. This means that you may not necessarily get answers to the questions you may have about the experience of visual impairment, but it does try to redress the balance of research activities which have been up until recently weighted to the curiosity of the sighted researcher as opposed to what visually impaired people think is important.

Narrative approaches to research

The use of narrative within social science research has been documented by researchers such as Richardson (1990; 2000); Ellis (1999) Ellis and Bochner (1992; 2000); Ellis and Flaherty (1992); Clandinin and Connelly (2000); Etherington (2000); Richardson Taylor et al. (2000); Langellier (2001); Reissman (2006). Oral history and life story projects have also used narratives to document the history and give voice to marginalised groups (Smith 1999; O'Neill and Harnindranath 2006; French et al. 2006; Cloke et al. 2000), and Pelias has spoken of how performance and arts based methods can be used to explore social processes (Pelias 1999) and indeed I, and others, have used narrative approaches to explore counselling processes (Dale 2010; Etherington 2000, 2001; Speedy 2007).

Within this book, narrative is used to "show" a dynamic process of research, through conversation, rather than a "telling" of a research process that has happened. The focus is firmly on the experience of visual impairment rather than a review of methodological approaches and conclusions. It uses narrative, specifically outsider witness practices (Myerhoff 1982) and definitional ceremony (White 2003) as a means to construct and convey identity.

I was introduced to outsider witness practices and definitional ceremony whilst studying narrative therapy as part of a Master of Science Counselling award. These practices and the phrase "definitional ceremony" were used initially by anthropologist Barbara Myerhoff to describe the way in which people could generate richer identity claims by telling stories of their life experiences and having these witnessed by others. For example people belonging to religious communities such as Jews or Christians (within worship ceremonies) tell the stories of God's relationship with people in the past to enable them to understand God's relationship with them here and now, and it is in the witnessing and sharing of these stories that people gain a sense of their own identity and worth. Sometimes however, as in the group of elderly Jewish people Myerhoff was working with, the natural occasions for this kind of witnessing did not happen, and individuals became increasingly isolated and the community fragmented.

> "when cultures are fragmented and in serious disarray, proper audiences may be hard to find. Natural occasions may not be offered and then they must be artificially invented. I have called such performances 'definitional ceremony'" (Myerhoff 1982:105).

Witnesses were not asked to "evaluate" the stories they heard (either in terms of praise or criticism, but rather to allow the stories to resonate with their own life experiences and the stories from their own lives that were evoked. These practices have been developed by Narrative therapists such as White and Epston (1990), Payne (2000) for use within their therapeutic practices and developed also by researchers such as Speedy (2007; 2004).

Isolation is one of the commonest "issues" cited by people with a visual impairment (Burmedi et al. 2002; Stephens 2007), and the opportunity to "witness" in this sense to each other is limited by the fact that people who are blind are a minority, and the practicalities of living with low vision means we often have to rely on others to facilitate meetings. Also, there is often the expectation from sighted communities that people who are visually impaired should be integrated into a sighted society rather than meet with each other. One manager at a local society for the blind responded to my suggestion of a support group for people affected by sight loss said,

> "we don't want to start a blind ghetto here, you never know what they might get up to if they meet in groups! The need is for them to become part of our community not a separate one".

What I discovered when I started to present or published stories about people's experiences of living with a visual impairment to audiences of blind and partially sighted people was that stories evoked stories. When stories were told those listening talked about; how what they had heard evoked strong feelings linked to their own experiences and they in turn told me stories about their own experiences. When I relayed these new stories to the original storytellers they expressed feelings of their experiences being validated, and felt a strong connection to these others.

Through the process of the telling of stories, these being witnessed by others who in turn have told their own stories there has been movement from individual fragmented voices to a collection of linked stories that are presented in this book.

There has been a growth within feminist traditions of what is described as "collective biography" which is as Speedy states: "work that draws the memories that people hold to in their lives through a process of telling, re-telling, writing and re-writing stories" (Speedy 2005:31) and through the re-telling and writing "reveal the ways in which we were (and are) collectively produced" (Davies et al. 2001:169). This book is not a "collective biography" (Davies et al. 2001) in the sense that the stories are not written collectively, with individual stories distilled into one collective voice, but they are a collection of stories connected across shared themes, thus instead of the process being one of reduction, the opposite occurs; many voices are added which give thick rich descriptions (White and Epston 1990) of a subject matter that is often thought of in very narrow terms. Our sense of community is being re-membered (White 1995). There is what White (1999) describes as "commutas – that unique sense of being present to each other in entering liminal circumstances, betwixt and between known worlds" and out of the unknown is born something new.

The narrative is presented as a tapestry of voices which challenge the privilege of medical and academic knowledge and will hopefully inspire other people who live with a visual impairment to tell of their experiences. The book is set out in three parts:

Part 1 Transitions will set the scene, introduce the contributors and include themes relation to transition from sighted to visually impaired. Chapter One "Diagnosis to Registration explores the experiences of being diagnosed with an incurable eye condition, and the journey from diagnosis through treatment possibilities, to losing sight and registration and includes part one of the commentary "the etiquette of the sighted". Chapter Two "Living with incurable sight loss" explores the experience of losing sight, in terms of emotion and practical issues that arise in daily living. It also includes part two of the commentary "the etiquette of the sighted". Chapter Three "Changing Relationships" focuses on how the dynamics of personal relationships change with loss of sight, and includes part three of the commentary "the etiquette of the sighted". Chapter Four "Employment, Study and Benefits" explores the experience of changing patterns in employment study and what living on benefits is like and includes part four of the commentary "the etiquette of the sighted" Chapter Five "Am I going Mad?" considers the experience of living with visual hallucinations and societal attitudes that link losing sight with deteriorating mental health. It includes a commentary that explores current literature relating to visual hallucinations and "Charles Bonnet Syndrome".

Part 2 – Living Life as someone who is blind or partially sighted; will consider the societal attitudes towards blindness and what it is like to live, long term, with limited vision in a world that values sight above all other senses. Chapter six "Societal attitudes towards blindness" explores how societal attitudes about visual impairment affect perceptions of self and identity. It includes the first part of commentary entitled "re-authoring blindness". Chapter Seven "Who am I if I cannot see you?" explores identity issues related to gender, sexuality and relationships and includes part two of the commentary "re-authoring blindness". Chapter Eight "Blindness and Disability Discrimination" explores how disabling practices have disempowered contributors and includes part three of the commentary "re-authoring blindness". Chapter Nine "New treatments, 'A step forward for humankind', or not?" explores whether visual impairment is always a medical condition that needs treatment or whether it is just a different way of being. It also includes part one of the commentary entitled "living in the twilight zone". Chapter Ten "Differences between blindness and partial sight" explores from different perspectives the experience of blindness and partial sight and includes part two of the commentary "living in the twilight zone".

Part 3 – Enabling practices and transforming identities considers how people's negative experiences of living with visual impairment can be minimised. Emotional support, counselling and emancipatory research practices are explored and how people can support themselves and enable dialogue with sighted professionals in ways that promote enabling rather than disabling practices. Chapter Eleven "Emotional Support" considers the emotional support needs of those who are losing sight and includes part one of the commentary entitled "developing emotional support services for people who are visually impaired". Chapter Twelve "Tales from the Counselling Room" explores contributor's experiences of using formal counselling and other psychological interventions and includes part two of commentary "developing emotional support services for people who are visually impaired". Chapter Thirteen "Joined up Voices" uses excerpts from group conversations between people who are blind and partially sighted to explore what moves them from feeling isolated, marginalised and without a voice to a vibrant community who have a degree of control over services.

Chapter Fourteen "Narrative Perspectives on Research" explores the use of narrative research practices to research the experience of living with a visual impairment and the impact of the research project on contributors. It also includes part two of the commentary "emancipatory research practices. Finally there is an Epilogue which is entitled "The re-grilling of Mr B".

Terminology

I have used the descriptions "blind or partially sighted" or "visually impaired" interchangeably to mean someone who is registered as either seriously sight impaired (blind) or sight impaired (partially sighted). I have also used the terms counselling, therapy, and psychotherapy interchangeably to mean a therapeutic undertaking agreed upon by someone who is commonly called a client and someone who is called counsellor, therapist, or psychotherapist.

Poetic representation

Representing conversation as text is always challenging, and much has been written on this subject for example within the works of Richardson (1992; 2000; 2003; 1990; 2000). We do not normally speak in the formal language of prose, but in what has been described by Tedlock (1983) as "dramatic poetry". I have therefore - as others have before me (Richardson 2003; Speedy 2005; Etherington 2000) presented conversation in stanza format. For a fuller discussion of my use of stanza format and how conversation is turned into text see Dale (2010) where a full discussion and examples of the process are included.

Introduction to contributors

Some contributors have chosen to use pseudonyms others have preferred to make contributions under their own names, they have all been part of the editorial process, but following consultation I have taken most of the decisions about what material to use and where to put it. Some contributors have been involved with the research project since 2005, others have joined the journey in the intervening years. Some have written much and others only a little. All their contributions however big or small have been valued and are, I consider, the vital element of the book which you are about to read.

All the contributors introduce themselves in ways they feel appropriate, and tell you the reader what they would like you to know about them, possibly not always what you would have chosen to ask! Their ages range from 22-89 years. All are registered as either sight impaired (partially sighted) or severely sight impaired (blind). Some have lost sight relatively recently others have always lived with a level of visual impairment. Sixteen are male fourteen are female. Most have varying degrees of residual vision, three have no vision at all. They are all developing a voice.

In alphabetical order they are: Adam, Andy, Ann, Anna, Annie, Beth, Caroline, Chris, Claire, Dennis, Emma, George, Jane, Maria, Martin, Matt, Maureen, May, Michael, Mike, Mo, Patrick, Pauline, Phil, Peter, Ray, Sarah, Stephen, Tony and Will.

PART 1

TRANSITIONS

CHAPTER ONE

DIAGNOSIS TO REGISTRATION

Sue: Journal February 23rd 2007

Coming home from work on the train on a cold day in February 2007 May's words rattled round in my mind and I write them (as much as I can remember) in my notebook. These notes were May's current description of her life, and are the backdrop against which our future conversations took place. It started me thinking about the way in which people are diagnosed, treated and then registered as either sight impaired (partially sighted) or severely sight impaired (blind) and the ways in which these moments often defined people within "thin problem saturated descriptions" (White and Epston 1990) that were difficult to escape from, and little support was offered to enable psychological adjustment or hope for the future.

May says of herself[1]:

> I sometimes think I have lived too long;
> I was well up to my late 70's,
> never had even a twinge.
> Then everything fell apart at the same time.

> This is not living,
> **it is just enduring**

> I coped with the arthritis,
> the Parkinson's,
> losing my son (that was the most awful time),
> even the cancer.
> But losing my sight is the **biggest insult**;
> being looked after like a baby!

> I've always had my pride.
> The **shame** of it.
> I am just a "blind woman" now
> I even have a certificate to prove it!

---

[1] My conversations with May were initially published in the article "The Grilling of Mr B: Using the narrative therapy practice of 'externalising' conversations to co-research the experience of blindness" Therapy Today 2009. 20 (7) and are reproduced here with permission.

"Blindness" is a real bugger!

In my conversations with many people who are visually impaired the starting point is often their descriptions of diagnosis and registration and these are often recalled and remembered vividly; perhaps in the way that people often remember a loved one's death, or where they were when J.F. Kennedy was assassinated, or when the planes crashed into the twin towers on 9/11.

The experience of these moments are often recalled with emphasis on "where I was, who I was with, what they said to me, how they or I behaved" and often linked with feelings of acute anxiety, despair, anger, disbelief and isolation, followed by depression. This ties in with research such as (Burmedi et al. 2002; Douglas, Pavey, and Corcoran 2008; Stephens 2007; Thurston 2010) where the points of diagnosis and registration are highlighted as key moments when people report feeling particularly anxious and depressed.

They are perhaps moments and turning points in life which come unwanted and unasked for, and are often delivered in ways that are not always helpful or supportive.

A journey into conversation

Dennis: A journey

　　Sue: into conversation

Dennis: thinking about
untreatable sight loss.

"there's nothing I can do
I don't need to book another appointment
I'm sorry but I've got a busy clinic.
Can you go now."

I know they don't say that
but that is what they imply.

　　Sue: That was the implication I heard
　　When I was sitting
　　talking to this very eminent professor.
　　Him saying:
　　"there is nothing we can do
　　so we can discharge you"-
　　That's it.

Such a sweeping statement.

Sue: Still left wondering,
"what are they telling me?"

They were purely focusing on "you" as an eye condition.
Not "you" as a person
and how it may impact.

Dennis: I'm just remembering my diagnosis
He said three things:
"There's nothing can be done
you've got macular degeneration".
Why not?
"YOU won't go completely blind".
   What the flippin heck does that mean?
   Can you explain?
   and you've used that word
BLIND!

"You must make provision for the future".
   At the time, I couldn't even think,
   I had my wife and a two-year-old baby
   sitting in the room with me.

   How the flippin hell do I do that?

How do I make provision for a future which you've just told me is going to
   be
damaged permanently by loss of sight?

That was the one that made me
more angry than any..

Literally was:
"I won't need to see you again".

   Sue: Goodbye!

Dennis: I don't think it was insensitive
But don't think it was necessarily friendly
It was just ..
Professional.

The etiquette of the sighted (Part One)

One of the comments that has touched me most relating to blindness was spoken by Andy (an ex-counselling client). He said, "we have to live within the etiquette of the sighted" (Dale 2008c:25). He was speaking of the ways in which people communicate using eye contact, body language and facial expression which were lost to him as a person with partial sight. He wanted to, "run my fingers over their faces and bodies to see who they were" but to do so would break social rules of etiquette, so in conforming to these rules he was deprived of the means to understand using other senses. Kinash says:

> "If you are sighted, close your eyes and what do you see? You see darkness. Try to walk around and attend to daily life and you are disoriented and crash into things. This is not the blind person's experience" (Kinash 2005:1).

95% of people who are registered as blind or partially sighted have some residual vision (RNIB 2008), so although many of us are registered as "blind", or are referred to, or refer to themselves as "blind", only a very small number of people have no vision or light perception at all. It is also worth remembering that even those with no vision at all do not see darkness, (Kinash 2005) but nothing.

The general public's perception of blindness or visual impairment, however, is often that those who use a white cane or a guide dog live in permanent darkness, and are either to be pitied and patronised, or, we are some kind of super-hero. People who are blind and partially sighted are in fact just that, people, they are not a homogenous group "the blind" but all have different levels of residual vision, and unique perceptions of what their visual impairment means to them, for some this is a positive experience, for others it is not.

Adam Hahn is an artist whose grandmother had macular degeneration (MD). Following a detailed interview with Dennis, who also has MD and is registered blind, Adam painted a picture, shown here with Dennis alongside, depicting a typical image of one of the main MD symptoms – the inability to recognise people:

> "By representing the person as they would see themselves these paintings engage the viewer in trying to understand how other people see" (Hahn 2008).

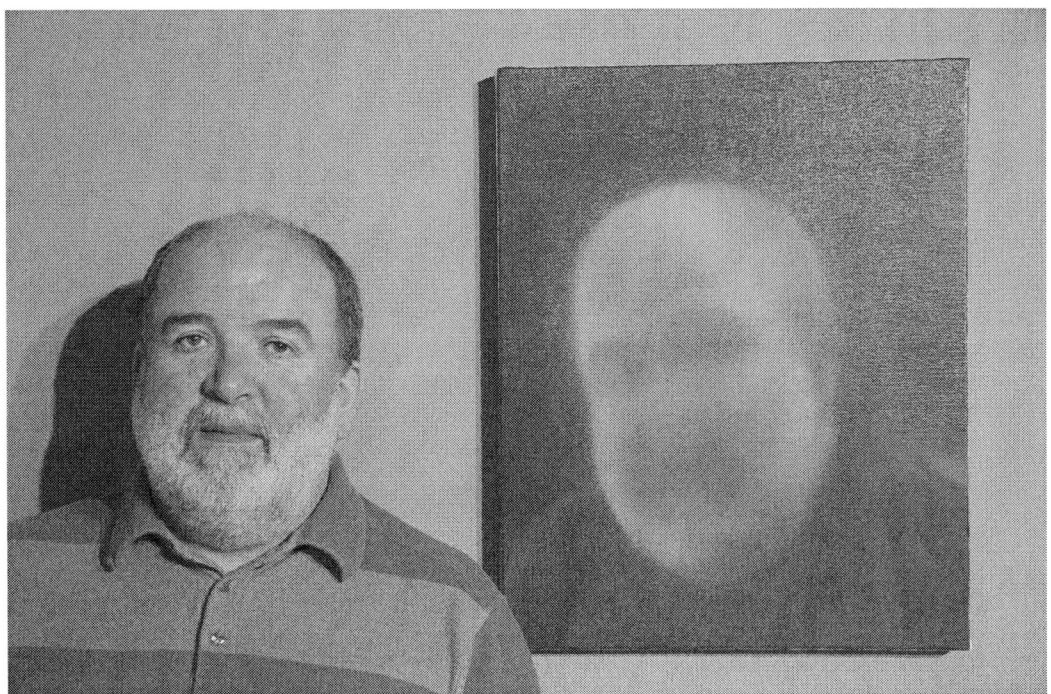

As I look at this portrait, especially this image with the photo of Dennis alongside his view of himself; "the before and after" as Dennis laughingly tells me. I find myself moved to tears mainly I think because I realise that it is so hard to understand someone else's experience of vision and what this might mean to them. The portrait is beautiful, ethereal, but as I look at both images, there is also a huge sense of difference and loss, one which I can not ever fully comprehend, because my vision has always been the same.

If I were to draw a portrait of what I see when I look in the mirror, it would be very different. The only time I see my whole face (or Dennis's for that matter) is when I look at a photograph where the image is small enough for me to see it all at once. I have not lost the ability to see detail, but I only see fragmented parts of a face, and as I shift my gaze I gradually build up a full picture.

Because of the peculiarities of my sight people often respond to me with confusion, I can be sitting on the train, working on my computer, apparently seeing quite well, and then on leaving the train having to get out my white cane to negotiate unfamiliar landscapes. "It's disgusting!" One woman said to her friend. "**She** can see as well as me. I've seen her on the train reading". Although someone voicing this opinion within my hearing is unusual, I am sure that it is the unvoiced opinion of many who do not know me well. The other side of the coin is that people often offer me sympathy rather than empathy with comments such as, "I didn't know about your sight, I am so very sorry", what I wonder are they sorry about? My sight is just part of who I am, and I am happy with it (well most of the time!). Or as an acquaintance said recently; "You are so amazing, managing to study to the level you do, with your disability". Why should that be so amazing? I am just ordinary, doing what thousands have done before me, and indeed this woman also has a masters degree! Is she amazing too?

Others join the journey

The stories emerging from my doctoral project between 2006 and 2009 created much interest amongst visually impaired audiences who accessed them through my presentations at various national and international conferences and training courses and also through reading the drafts of various journal articles (Dale 2008c; 2009a; 2008a). and listening to the stories included in the audio dissertation produced for my doctorate (Dale 2009b). These audiences did not respond with critical reviews, or learned thesis, but with further stories of their own life experiences. New narratives were emerging told out through email, telephone, and face to face contact. These new narratives were giving a "thick rich description" (White and Epston 1990) of the experience of living with a visual impairment.

> Email received from Michael:
> Hi Sue
> Is diagnosis with an incurable eye condition the beginning, the end of the beginning, or the beginning of the end?

He emailed me following a presentation that I had given at a national vision conference. He had been listening to an audio clip where Sarah described her experience of being diagnosed with MD (Macular Disease):

> **Sarah[2]**
> I'm 58 quite assertive normally
> I can't believe how the hospital told me
> Can't believe it.
> Even sitting here telling you
> I think that I must have imagined it.
>
> "She's got MD" he said to the student.
> "There is no hope of recovery the retina is damaged beyond repair"
> Still they didn't talk to me.
>
> I blink slowly.
> "what does this mean for me?" I ask

---

[2] Sarah's story was originally published as part of article "Knitting in the dark: narratives about the experience of sight loss in a counselling session" in British Journal of Visual Impairment September 2008 and is included here with permission.

"We'll make an appointment to get you registered"
He said,
"you don't have to worry about it".

What! Me! Worry!

Then I was out in the street.
Should I drive home?
Did I really hear what they said?
If I couldn't drive….
I started shaking then.
Uncontrollably.
I didn't know where the bus went from.

Michael went on to say:

Diagnosis did not come as a shock to me, although it was shocking. In some ways it was a relief, because I now knew what was going on, and in other ways it felt like a death sentence. I'd been having problems with my eyes for the best part of a year, had been to numerous ophthalmic clinics, waited hours in varying corridors, had huge amounts of tests, drops, people peering into my eyes.

Lots of fear, hope, anger, despair… a rollercoaster of emotions!

When he said the words "Retinitis Pigmentosa (RP), degenerative, no treatment possibilities at present" they felt imprinted in my brain. Like Sarah I couldn't believe what I was hearing. Sat like a rabbit in the headlights.

I don't know whether he told me in a caring way or whether the nursing staff were helpful even. I really can't remember. I was in shock. I went out of the door a print out from the computer in my hand about RP and no further appointment booked. I sat on the bench by outpatients and wept. I just didn't know what would become of me.

Registration was different. That came later when I was struggling at work. That just left me feeling written off. A full stop. A certificate ending my life as a sighted person. I felt angry; with the world, with God, with people who had 20/20 vision – with everybody.

I spent hours looking carefully at photos, places I loved, my children's faces imagining a world one day when I wouldn't see them, and then the anger and despair came.

I really didn't want to be there!

I visited Annie at home. She had telephoned me to arrange a visit after hearing the audio version of Sarah's story whilst on a course at the RNIB.

Annie: I want to tell you about my experiences" she said "because I
really think that this may help change what it is like for people like
me....
I always go to the eye hospital with my daughter,
my husband hates it and I don't want to go alone.

Being diagnosed has happened in bits and pieces,
one bit of the problem followed by another
and always the prognosis gets worse.

It has involved going to hospital, like I did yesterday

I sit and wait
like a thousand times I have before
I hold in my hand the number..
When you arrive you have to take a ticket
          just like at the deli counter in Sainsbury's

When a voice calls out
          Number 68 (your time is up!)
you make your way to the window
          if you can see where it is!
then they get out your file, put it in a basket on the left and
ask you to sit on the red chairs.
          If you can see them,
you do.

Then you wait.

And wait

Staff rush about talking madly
people like me line the chairs

and we wait

"Tomkins...."

A disembodied voice

"Tomkins"

          Louder this time
"This way please"
I follow if I can see where!

The nurse sits me in a chair
          "cover your left eye dear and read the chart from the top"
I do if I can see it!
Failure always seizes me in the silences.

Drops are administered
to dilate the pupils
"wait now on the blue chairs"

I wait,
        and wait.

"Tomkins"
        says a voice eventually

I sit in the black chair
The man hoovers up my eyes with the machine.
The questions begin.

His breath brushes my face
        "look left... up...down"
I am pressed against the head and chin rest.
My neck cricks and creaks

He retreats,
there is silence.
He writes
I wait.

I have done this a thousand times before it seems.
But it was only 6 months ago the optician said to me
"I don't like the look of this – we'll need to get you seen at the
hospital."
Now the words hover in the air.
As well as glaucoma I have untreatable cataracts.

May speaks to me following my request for permission to include
her story in an article in a counselling journal (Dale 2009) and says
about registration:

May: The certificate that sealed my fate as a blind woman
was given to me by the hospital.
It is all that I am now
BLIND
I couldn't read it though
the print was too small!

What's the use of that?"

Andy also talks of his interaction with the eye clinic:

Andy: [3]She –at the hospital- told me that living without sight

---

[3] Andy's story was first presented by me at the International Conference
of Narrative Therapy and Community Work in Norway 2007, the written
version appearing as part of article "Knitting in the dark: narratives about

doesn't have to be a tragedy
that I can go on and have a "fulfilling life"!
that I need to put a "brave face on it"
and I do – I think.
What the hell does she know though?
She doesn't live my life.
She just wants me to say I'm ok
so that she can feel better about it all!

I can't do this.

I don't want to.

I think about dying sometimes
it seems like a kind of relief to think
that it will all end one day.

Presenting this and other stories at national and international conferences and talking about the process of diagnosis and registration elicits further emails:

Email from Matt
Hi Sue,
Thank you for your words in Norway.
Do you think that being registered makes any difference? I was registered as blind years ago, and apart from a free TV license, a white cane and a talking watch it hasn't got me very much or very far!

The hospital who delivered the verdict signed me off. Rather like receiving your P45 stating "unemployable".

Perhaps registration is so that the sighted remember who we are before they ignore us!!

I have conversations with Peter:

Peter: After listening to your talk in Birmingham I started to think about my own experiences in a different way.

I started to think that being diagnosed, and registered, and how people help you then is key to how you cope when your sight goes.
Because what I experienced,
and others that I have talked to have said,
is that the hospital builds up such a lot of stress
and puts so much emphasis on treatment
and what they can do,
that when they can't...

---

the experience of sight loss in a counselling session" in British Journal of Visual Impairment September 2008 and is included here with permission.

When they have to finally say
"there is nothing more we can do"
and you don't go there any more
It feels like

failure...

That you have failed,
and you're a "write off"
Like the car when the repairs cost too much to get through the MOT.

Then you are left.
No one checks to see how you're coping,
if you're lucky you might see the social worker who'll give you a
watch and a symbol cane..

But that's it.

It would have really helped if someone had been there for me to talk
to.
Even my family talked to me as if I was an idiot
they didn't know how to cope with me.

They wanted me to go into a home.
But I wouldn't.

Now, the diagnosis doesn't really matter.
It's just a label...
Not really me at all.

Participants in Thurston's (2010) study commented on their experiences of being diagnosed and these tie in very much with the experiences of contributors to this book. One says:

"I went out at nine o'clock in the morning quite hale and hearty and I came back at night unable to drive and registered as disabled at my work. Nobody said here's a leaflet or information on anything else. I came back and I didn't know if I was going to be blind in six months and it was really traumatic and it could have been a lot less traumatic" (Thurston 2010:6)

How the person is dealt with at the times of diagnosis and registration seems to have a critical bearing on how quickly they have adjusted to living with their visual impairment. As Thurston points out:

"During diagnosis patients need to make sense of the diagnosis of sight loss on three levels – intellectually, practically and emotionally. Clinicians can help by trying to satisfy this need on all three levels. At present, this does not seem to be happening, with patients complaining particularly about lack of information and a perceived lack of care during the time of diagnosis". (ibid:6)

Stephen emails me:

Hi Sue
I have been recently diagnosed with proliferative diabetic retinopathy and told that I will eventually go blind. I have been a diabetic and insulin dependent for many years, and have fought battles with my body as long as I can remember.

This diagnosis however is the hardest thing I have ever had to bear. It feels like this is the final straw, not seeing affects every part of life, takes away my dignity and my courage to go on.

I think how the news was delivered did not help. It was a busy clinic. I had been waiting for at least 2 hours. I was finally ushered into the presence of the consultant. He had two students with him. All of them examined my eyes. They had a conversation between themselves about the recent laser treatment and the amount of scar tissue. Then looking briefly up from the notes he said "I don't think there's any point in any further treatment, it will not make any difference. I'm sorry. We'll see you again in 12 months to see how things have changed. Your visual acuity means that I will if you wish register you as severely sight impaired (blind) and make an appointment for you to see the social worker who will tell you what kinds of benefits you could be entitled to".

I felt as if I couldn't understand what he was saying, even though he was speaking in plain English. I had been going backwards and forwards to the hospital every month for at least a year, and they had been giving me regular laser treatment, now they were saying they were giving up on me. Giving me up for what? Where did I go now? Surely with all these new treatment possibilities there was something that could be done? Perhaps new glasses would help?

There was such a lot of fear, like stepping off the edge of the world, and I didn't much like the look of the world that I was falling into.

My wife who was with me said that she wasn't altogether surprised, that they had talked about this before, she tried to reassure me it wouldn't make any difference. I couldn't remember them talking about it before, or perhaps I didn't want to hear what they were saying. Somehow up until that moment there was hope and now it had gone. I was so angry, disappointed. What good was registration going to be? It couldn't bring my sight back.

Jane emails me having read some of the publications relating to my study. She was interested in contributing to the proposed book.

Dear Sue

I wrote this the other day with your book in mind. However, it's my first run through and very much how I felt at the time. Sometimes I need to write something down to find out how I feel. If I wrote it again, it would be very different. I'm sending you a copy but will probably write something else soon. Writing in itself, is therapeutic!

Where does one Start?

Where does one start? Fumbling around sums up how my life is at the moment. From being an independent, capable self-sufficient woman, I'm struggling to find my place in society. My identity has changed dramatically, along with the inability to see.

I suffer with Dystonia, a condition which causes uncontrollable spasms in certain focalised areas of the body. Mine is a form called Blepharospasm, which causes involuntary spasms around the eyes. They are so severe that my eyes are closed for at least 80% of the time. This renders me functionally blind. I would be able to see if I could physically open them.

Typically, this came upon me gradually at around 55 years of age. (I've since learnt that the average age of onset is 55 years.) I had chronic Dry Eye with my left eye weeping constantly.

I attended the Eye Clinic at my local hospital after having tried various drugs prescribed by my GP to stop the spasms. I had already stopped driving so took a taxi. My name was called and I tried to follow the disappearing consultant. Not being able to see, I had no idea where he'd gone to. I also careered into a low coffee table inconveniently positioned in the middle of the floor. This was an eye clinic for goodness sake!

He was most insistent that I open my eyes. I desperately tried and was able to flicker them open and stare ahead whilst he examined me. He got very frustrated because I couldn't keep them open. He prescribed drops to lubricate them. Nothing more. So what about not being able to see? Does that not matter? Will the drops stop the spasms? My turn was up so I was discharged from the clinic. Was that it?

I sobbed whilst waiting for the taxi. Where were the answers? What was wrong with me? I was fed up with struggling, stuck in the house. I kept bumping into door frames, walls getting caught on door handles. I was helpless and vulnerable. Was I mad? How would I know?

My husband cut his hours at work because I needed so much help round the house. I couldn't drive, shop, and simple things like carry two glasses of water. I needed to feel my way around the house. My co-ordination was also shot. I gauged distances by looking briefly as my eyes flicked open. I advanced with relative confidence only to veer off into walls or doorframes. Who moved them?!

I was used to attending an aqua class at the local swimming pool twice a week. It was winter and I recall leaving the changing room, making for the pool. I'd forgotten to take off a T-shirt I wore as a vest. I burst into tears once I was told. How humiliating! On another occasion, I was having a conversation with the class teacher. Suddenly, the woman next to me told me that she'd gone. I was addressing thin air! This was before I'd acknowledged the problem and told folk I needed help. Since then, they've been fabulous. Admitting that I wanted help was hard though. At the time, I didn't have a white stick or a signal cane. As far as the hospital was concerned, I could see fine! Trouble was, I couldn't open my eyes.

Working as a counsellor and knowing about the body's ability to express what we can't verbalise, I was concerned that my condition might be psychosomatic. I had a dog that had lost his sight. I wondered if I was empathising with him. I had tried acupuncture, now I wanted to try hypnotherapy. If I was somehow causing this, maybe I could also cure it!

I fought for a referral to an ENT specialist, convinced there must be something simple wrong with me. He found nothing wrong with me but suggested I saw a neurologist. Again, I had to fight for an appointment. Was I costing the NHS too much money?

The local neurologist that I saw immediately diagnosed Blepharospasm. What a relief! This weird and not so wonderful twitching had a name! So how do I get better? Learning that there was treatment, even though this was a life long condition, didn't seem too bad. He injected me straight away with either Dysport or Botox. I was waiting for the miracle to happen – my eyes to open. They didn't.

In the meantime, I turned to our local Visual Impairment Team. I realise that all this research I had to do myself. Finding help was extremely difficult. However, through them I received training in walking with a white stick. I felt unsure using it at first. I thought my husband would be embarrassed taking out a woman who was not only functionally blind but also having ugly, uncontrollable, facial spasms. I needed to feel the sunlight on my face. It's still not my favourite activity but I'll do it if necessary. If I don't, I'm trapped in the house. It would be so easy to hide away.

From my local hospital, I was sent to a London Hospital. Again I was treated here for nearly two years without success. They told me that they were experts. They were my last port of call. "The buck stops here".

I had injections every three to four months. The spasms were a little less apparent for about a month then returned with a vengeance. I was told that other patients responded well to this. What was wrong with me then? Was I causing it? Was I a mad?

I've tried taping my eyes open. They are so sore. The spasms are so strong that the tape doesn't hold them open completely for longer that about 20 minutes. I have isolated myself to such an extent that when I was invited to a wedding, I felt I had to try. I used to be so gregarious, able to mingle, put people at their ease. My husband and I sat alone for most of the evening. I'd taped my eyes open but really couldn't see for much of the time. I thought I looked crazy. I was having facial spasms. No wonder no one came near us. I could have screamed. THIS IS NOT ME!!!! Trying to put a brave face on afterwards was impossible. I sobbed.

I ordered some ptosis props to attach to my glasses, metal bars that supposedly hold the eyes open. They don't! I also have FL41 tints to ease the glare. I wear cocoons bought from RNIB over my ordinary glasses but am still very sensitive.

Through the Dystonia Society and my own Internet searches, I read about another specialist in another hospital. Now I had a diagnosis, my GP was more amenable to ask for a second opinion. This specialist thought she could do better than the previous one. She was quite honest saying that the proof was in the pudding.

Three days after her injections, my eyes were wide open! I couldn't shut them but I didn't care! The world looked as though it were in colour. I could do things again.

Unfortunately, the first treatment didn't last longer than a month. The second lot was less successful. But, the remedy is in adjusting the dosage and sites to fit me. I have faith. There are worse things in life and I must adjust to this variable condition. Let's hope that next time works better!

This is the first chapter of the book, a starting point, and as you read the accounts people have written you will notice how these change over time and as the chapters progress. What we write is true at the time, but the process of writing, and the passage of time means we write ourselves into somewhere or someone different.

Sue: Journal October 2007
Coming back from work on the train I think more about the conversations that I have had with people and how diagnosis and registration seem to catapult the person into a different world. Rather like my memories of watching the TV series "Star Trek" with my son and seeing Mr. Spock being transported from a spaceship into a distant land full of aliens.

Entering the world of the visually impaired is not what many people would want to do. As Rebecca Atkinson points out of her experience of moving from being sighted to being blind, "You are about to cross over into the dark side and see what wriggles and writhes on the under belly of society. Folk will see you as the sufferer, the pitiful, the afflicted, the subhuman – that's you, yes, you" (Atkinson 2007). It is a world where there are very negative images of being dependent, a victim and the experience is isolating.

After all at the hospital when you are diagnosed and registered the sighted people around you are all employed, and all rush about looking efficient and busy, and the blind and partially sighted line the corridors on plastic chairs unable to see even each other! And if you are one of those sitting on the chairs, then the process is out of your control.

Chapter Two

Living with Incurable Sight Loss

Within this chapter I intend to reflect on the diversity of response to living with a visual impairment and engage the reader with the second part of a commentary considering the "etiquette of the sighted". There is an exploration of the experience of losing sight, in terms of the emotion of losing a sense, practical issues that arise in daily living, the challenges of rehabilitation and having to learn new ways of doing things and finally responses to these stories from people who have lived with a visual impairment for many years.

__Journal September 2008__
Useless
I didn't see the stone,
I felt the pain of it,
the sting as it caught my face,
"you're useless you blind binch"
(Rolf wasn't very literate even with his swearing!).
I held my ground,
feet planted firmly apart,
my chin thrust forward,
a show of bravado,
but...
inside...
I wanted to die.
I was 6,
maybe 7
We had been playing "can"
a team game where stones were thrown towards a can,
and the team with the most hits was the winner.
But I missed.
I always missed.
That word __again..__
__Useless.__

It followed me like a curse,
through school,
not home,
there I was a "beautiful princess"
according to my father,

but that didn't tie in with how others saw me.
I became a withdrawn teenager,
'Susan is a quiet child who tags along with the rest, but works hard'
'tries hard but finds it difficult to keep up, not really academic' were
reports that repeated.

As stated earlier, there is often an assumption from sighted people about what blindness means. Often responses to sight loss and visual impairment are spoken about in terms of models related loss and bereavement. There is an expectation that a person who is visually impaired will go through a process of grieving for something that is lost, going through a series of feelings including sadness anger and depression and finally there will be an adjustment to life without sight. In practice however although grief and feelings of sadness, depression and anger are often present, especially for someone who has lived as sighted person all their life then loses some or all of their vision, the model is far too simplistic and does not take into consideration that visual impairment is a generic term which covers a multitude of different conditions which all affect individuals uniquely. To give you a personal example: walking to a restaurant one evening with Dennis I am aware of the differences in our experiences of this seemingly simple event. I have no peripheral or night vision, so negotiating the unfamiliar streets of London is extremely difficult for me. I take Dennis's arm and he alerts me to road crossings and potential hazards such as lampposts and wheelie bins which litter the pavements. When we arrive at the restaurant the menu arrives. Dennis has reduced central vision so cannot access the menu without the use of his monocular, my central vision is relatively fine so I read the menu. Our evening then continues uninterrupted. Visual impairment has had an effect on both of us, but in totally different ways. Things I find a problem he finds relatively easy and visa versa.

To explore some of these different responses let us firstly consider what people who have recently been diagnosed with incurable sight loss have said to me:

Sarah: I look into the mirror – nothing just a fading out.
Like my life really.
Just fading out, ending, useless.
Did I ever think I knew about life and who I was.
I knew nothing.
Nothing.
I sit for hours just sitting
Thinking nothing.
What else is there to do
I can' t sew, I can' t read
I close my eyes and try to recall the words on the pages of Tolkien.

Seeing them clearly in my mind gives me comfort.
Sitting with my eyes closed I can daydream, see colour and faces
I open my eyes and the world fades backwards
The dream world is preferable to this.

Each night I pray that I won't wake up.
But I always do.
It's always the same just at that moment of waking.
Hope then despair.

Martin emails me following a presentation of Sarah and Andy's stories at a conference:

Hi Sue,
About a year ago the diabetes which I had lived with for years claimed most of my vision, and I was registered as blind.

I remember my life sometimes, the life I had when I was a sighted person. It is like looking at a life that belonged to someone else that I can vaguely remember. Losing my sight has been like losing a loved one, no, not a loved one; it is more about losing the life that I loved and the person I was, and becoming someone else not of my choosing. An alien, trapped in an alien body that I cannot even see. There is something so different about navigating the world from a "seeing" perspective, than not being able to see where I am in relation to anyone else. People told me that my other senses would compensate. They never did, and they never will, in fact I think my hearing has got worse, probably because when we listen we pick up a lot of clues as to what is going on from our vision.

I grieved, I still grieve for my life that was. On the surface I cope well, but deep down I mourn my death.

Both Sarah and Martin lost sight over a relatively short period of time, but this is not always the case. Often people lose sight over many months or years, their condition is degenerative, so each day, or week or year there are new losses, there is an ongoing relationship with the eye clinics and treatment possibilities. Pauline talks about her experience of living with a combination of glaucoma and cataracts:

Pauline: It's worse again.
Even Worse.

My son gets cross, says it can't possibly be getting even worse
because I have been saying this for years.
But **it is worse**.

I feel so disconnected from everyone.
I can't seem to feel part of anything anymore,

even in one-to-one situations where I am sitting directly opposite the
person.
I feel trapped in my own world.
Totally trapped,
and that keeps getting worse.

What am I going to do?
It keeps getting worse and I can see even less
I'm so afraid….
It's been going on for so long.

I look at my granddaughter playing in the garden,
how long will I still be able to see her face?

A good Nan would be able to read to her.
I can't now
A good Nan would be able to look after her for the weekend
to give my daughter in law a break.
What use am I?
But it's more than that,
If it keeps getting worse what will it mean for me?
Who will I be when I can't see my granddaughters face?
Each time they try something new at the hospital I get my hopes up.
Then they are dashed.
The result is usually worse.
Even worse.

The older I get the more afraid I am,
of not coping,
of having to go into a home.
Of being useless.

As people make their way through what is described as the "eye
care pathway" (RNIB) and their sight deteriorates they have to find
different ways of doing things. Mobility becomes problematic, tasks
related to employment or the home become more challenging.
People, both those losing their vision and those trying to engage
them in different ways of doing things (such as rehabilitation
officers) often tell me of ambivalent feelings regarding engaging
with these processes, especially the use of the white cane.

Andy[1] says:
"I use a white stick
I need it to feel my way through the streets
Like some kind of broken insect
Creeping round the ground
Tapping, poking, scratching, tasting.

---

[1] Part of Andy's story was included in an article which appeared in the
British Journal of Visual Impairment – see Dale 2008a for full details.

I need it, yet hate it.
How I hate it.

It represents everything I hate and despise
I have fantasises of smashing it, breaking it
hacking it into a hundred pieces and then burning it.

Burning it – seeing the flames lick it into dust.
Then scattering the ash to the wind.

People stand in the way
Make encouraging noises
The sweat trickles down my arms
Why do they stand in the way?
Stupid, stupid.
The silent watchers waiting for my slip.
The condescending murmurs of encouragement.

Finding my way now takes all my concentration
I find my way by learning the route.

I record in my mind every dip in the pavement
Each lamppost
Each fence
I physically reach out with my stick
Like a bomb disposal expert searching for mines
tap, tap, tap.
Never ever just walking and thinking about something else
Concentrating so hard.
I break out in a sweat
Someone stops me
I lose the plot
Where am I?
The person – afraid, backs off at my angry response.
I am alone.

Somehow losing my sight has changed all my senses
My body is constantly tense
Trying so hard to notice the least change of sound,
loss of vision makes it harder to hear to link in with others
I am so angry all the time
Angry bitter thoughts
consume me.

I live a lie
"I'm ok"
I tell my friend
"I'm coping well"
I've got a stick
And this guy who comes and tells me I'm doing ok
And I am.
I get out, walk the walk, talk the talk.

Stumble my way through pavements strewn with
bins, people, cars.
So cheerful – "well done" they cry

The lie kind of protects me
like the stick I suppose
moves people away from me
Being vulnerable is something I've always dreaded.

Reality though is that its shit.
I'm not ok.
I hate it.
I'll never accept it. (never? no never, never? well hardly ever – my
head bursts into a refrain from the pirates of Penzance)
Life isn't worth living.
But I live it because I'm too afraid not to.
I wish I didn't have to".

Rehabilitation services for people who are eligible for registration
as sight impaired or severely sight impaired differs from region to
region and is usually provided by the local authority or contracted
by them to local organisations or national charities. These days the
support is usually undertaken locally, one such team says:

"The RNIB South West Rehabilitation Services Team works with blind
and partially sighted people to enable them to enhance, retain or
develop independence. Where appropriate, residual vision is used to
re-establish old skills and acquire new ones. Rehabilitation may be
provided in either the user's home, the local environment or at the
RNIB South West Resource Centre, as appropriate.

Training areas covered include:
•   Independent living skills: information, advice and training in
the kitchen and other domestic tasks.
•   Orientation and mobility skills: indoors and out, to enable safe
and independent travel in relation to the person's sight loss. This
may include training with a cane and/or planning routes.
•   Communication skills: information, advice and training in a
wide variety of communication methods, including keyboard, braille
and Moon.
•   Demonstration of, and training with, specialised equipment,
including TV magnifiers.
•   Information on services and sources of advice within and
outside RNIB, eg Talking Books and Guide Dogs for the Blind". (RNIB
2010)

Annie says:
This nice young lady from the social came to see me,
she brought a gadget to help me make tea.
When you pour in the hot water and it gets near the top of the mug
it peeps so you know that you've poured in enough.

I put it in the cupboard.
Perhaps one day I might use it,
but I don't want to.

It was nice of her to come,
but not really what I want at all.
The only thing that would help would be improved vision
and they tell me that won't happen.

Prior to the emphasis on providing rehabilitation services to people within their own environment residential training was offered (and still is in some areas). Dennis talks about his experience in the 1980's of attending a residential rehabilitation course which was run by the RNIB in a specialist centre in Torquay.

Dennis: There were two houses,
the main house called Manor House,
and then there was also America Lodge,
and the people who went to America Lodge were the people that the staff and the system down there were satisfied that they could live independently.

So there was no rehab or carer support at America Lodge.
People,
visually impaired people,
would look after themselves,
but you couldn't get there,
they had to agree that you were eligible
so everyone that went there stayed in the main house,
and you were constantly monitored.
You didn't do anything,
every bit of food you ate was put in front of you
and the dirty stuff taken away.
Your washing;
you had to do your own washing,
but facilities were made for support with that,
and it was really a question of attending whatever classes you were going to
during the day,
and then in the evening the time was your own.

I can remember one or two individuals that were in a bit of a state,
not only physically,
but mentally,
and I think it would probably have been unsafe for them to go out by themselves.
I was thrown into that.

Sue: From being working in the bank, a professional environment for years and years..

What was interesting as well,
was at the bank,
because of the issues
that had arisen because of my sight problems
I felt I probably wasn't
just quite as good as anybody else anymore.

I couldn't do the job as quickly as other people,
and I was going through
all the things one goes through;
of not recognising people
and people saying things like,
"you just ignored me the other day"
"we passed each other in the office"
having to explain.
Or in the street,
or on the London Underground,
so that had made me feel that I wasn't quite as capable as most
people anymore,
and suddenly I find myself in Torquay
and I'm almost like top of the pile for
visually impaired people.
I've got a job for a start
and I have got macular disease;
which is central vision blindness
there were people there who had no vision.

So there was a lot of grief,
there was a lot of angst in the air in Torquay,
there was,
and I think that's what really
helped me sort my head out
because it helped me by seeing people
in all different stages of despair really.

And I remember one particular incident,
because I hadn't been there very long,
and the guy who was in the room with me
was the "house captain";
and if any of the people at the house
had problems with the staff ,
they would go to him and he would
represent them with staff
and that was quite structured,
I thought that was quite good!

He said to me one day,
"you know I have found our next house captain"
and I said, "who"
and he said "you".
And I said "well I don't know".

I said "I don't know,
I'm not sure about that, can I think about it?"
and he said, "okay".

And a couple of days later he approached me again
and he said,
"you know what I said?"
and I said yes, and he said,
"well actually
I have been talking with a few of the others
and I hope you don't mind,
but we are not sure it is a good idea".

I said, "Oh ok,
change of heart?

Do you mind if I ask what changed your mind?
He said,
"well,
we feel you are not typical of someone that's here,
you're not representative of the majority,
because the majority are out of work".

There were only one or two other people there that had families,
most of them were single people,
because of their eye problems
they were having difficulties
even just finding a partner.

Or finding someone to have fun with,
or to go out with
have a date.
Romance was ..

So consequently
because most of the people there were visually impaired there was a lot of
romance that went on.

What he said actually made sense
and I said,
"it's ok I'm not offended"

and I really wasn't offended,
"no its ok I do understand".
He'd seen this confident guy,
married,
got a job;
you know he should be able to represent people,
but he hadn't really thought through
the fact that people might say,
"it's alright for him he's got a job,

he's got a wife,
he's got kids..
I want all those,
so how does he know what if feels like to me".

So ..
that helped me just to get to know
how I was trying to cope with the condition.

Well that was where I first learnt to touch type.
Talking cube computers were in their early days,
but they were using them,
but they were a bit unscientific.

But I think the touch typing helped,
and because I had an office job,
the usual process that any person arriving at the centre would go
through in terms of assessing them,
I didn't go through that because
there were things like…,

there was a carpentry shop

They customized the course for me.
Yes that's right
and of course part of it
what everybody went through
I also went through
was the psychological side.

I would go out on mobility training,
and they would stick a blindfold on you
and help you familiarise yourself with using a guide cane;
not a symbol cane and …
that was interesting.
Well to be honest it never felt real.
It didn't feel real,
and I used to go out;
they'd take you round the streets of Torquay
and get you to cross roads ..
feel for obstacles on the pavement,
but all the time I'm thinking;
"what good is this to me?
From what I've been told about macular disease
I'm never going to be blind".

And another thing that everybody did
was learn to read Braille
that included me
and all I ended up doing
was looking at the dots with my magnifier.
(Laughter)

Sue: So you didn't go for the "touchy feely"?...

I couldn't ..
I tried the touchy feely bit,
and I couldn't do it..

Whether I'm clumsy or what,
I couldn't do it.
But in hindsight
thinking back
what is really interesting is..
I don't know who constructed the course
but there were just certain assumptions
made about blindness
that didn't apply to a lot of people.
Like I had a sight problem
but I'm not losing all of my sight.
And in fact the most comfortable people there
(although it sounds a bit crazy saying it)
were those that were totally blind!

Because they knew where they were at.
They knew exactly where they were at.
That's a horrible thought,
shutting your eyes and imagining;
that's what the rest of your life is going to be like.

Sue: But you if you know that's how it is then..

You either adjust,
or don't adjust.
But the majority of people
are in this partially sighted,
legally blind situation
and of course one tries to manage as best as one can.

Sue: so you're living in a almost kind of a twighlight world
I mean quite often I feel
I live in a kind of ..
I'm not one or the other

There were people at Torquay
who didn't want to go home.
It was quite sad really
because they had nobody at home
and here they had got support,
they got ready food,
they got pocket money.
You got pocket money.
I didn't get any because I was on a wage,
but most people were out of work

so they got whatever benefits were available
they were eligible for
and they also got some pocket money
and of course they'd go straight down the pub!

Often the loss of sight comes alongside other complications of old-age (The majority of people diagnosed with serious sight loss are over 65 years old). There are also often feelings of being a fraud, "I'm not really blind, I can see a bit" (Annie) and a reluctance to use the white cane. Mo says:

Mo: What me?
Use a white cane?
You must be joking!
I'd rather get run over than that.
I'm too old for all this malarkey!

Another issue spoken about frequently by people who lose vision in adulthood is the ability to drive. Giving up driving seems to represent something more than just swapping one transport system for another. The ability to drive seems intrinsically linked with identity and being as "an independent professional who can go places" (Caroline).

Michael emails with his views on what is difficult about being diagnosed with a visual impairment.

Hi Sue,
You asked me what the most difficult thing about being diagnosed with RP was, well there are lots! but I suppose the thing that instantly changed, other things have changed slowly along with my diminishing sight, but the one thing that changed instantly was not being able to drive. I was told at the time of my diagnosis that I would have to give up because my sight did not come up to the standards required.

This was devastating. I had always earned my living by driving, although in latter years I was more office bound, I had a company car, and a caravan, we used to spend our holidays journeying through Europe. Although my wife does drive, she really did not want to tow the caravan. It is strange but driving represented something about my manhood, my ability to be "somebody", I bought my first car (an elderly cortina) when I was 17, and was so proud. I had moved up in the world. The first time I went on the bus I sat with the mothers with young children, and the elderly ladies struggling with the shopping and thought "this is really the end". We lived out in the countryside so suddenly I couldn't get out, unless my wife took me, and that then limited her own activities, and did nothing for my feeling of being the man of the house. After a while work helped me get some access to work support and I was able to get a taxi to and from the train station, but in the end we had to move. I lost the house I had worked so hard to buy and then transform into a home.

Although my sight has always been poor I was not diagnosed with a visual impairment until my late twenties – I reflect here on how that affects me:

Sue: Journal October 2008
I learnt to drive at 17 –
Well everyone did where I lived in the country.
I was useless!
Nervous,
sick before lessons,
"Oh for God's sake … what is wrong with you?"
said my boyfriend,
"It's only a driving lesson,
just get on with it".

So I did.
After 39 lessons, and 2 failed tests
I sat in the car.
The examiner got in.
"Read that number plate over there"
he said without looking up.

I duly recited the letters.

I could see perfectly well in straight lines.

"Turn right out of the test centre" he said.
I felt sick. Panic consumed me.
The shame of feeling so scared took over.

"Come on"
he said kindly,
"It'll be alright!"

Turning right out of the centre he slammed on the brakes.
A bus was coming,
large,
"double deckered"
and red.

I hadn't seen it.

He thought it was nerves,
perhaps it was.

I took a deep breath,
and managed to negotiate the course,
without disgracing myself,

and to my surprise I passed.

This was the start of my life as a visually impaired driver,
(although at the time, I didn't know about the visual impairment)
I never looked back.

Well actually I had to look back a hundred times,
constantly scanning for traffic,
never sure,
It was just such hard work.

I thought this was what everybody did,
it was just they were good at it,
and I was...
Useless

One night,
it was my turn to drive back from the pub,
the others were giggling or asleep,
too much cider and black I suspect,
Marianne had to go back to Somersham.

Through the lanes I went.
Black,
Black,
blacker...
I slowed to a crawl,
then lost the road.
I don't know how.
But I was definitely in a field.
Should I alert my boyfriend?

No.

Shame held me back.

*He would say something like "you useless f****ing woman"*
and wrench the wheel out of my hand,
and he had drunk too much to drive anyway.

They hadn't noticed...
I crept round the field
keeping the wing mirror against the hedge,
until,
miraculously
we got back on the road.
I never told,
they never knew.

I was 17 then,
and it was not until 10 years later that I was diagnosed with CSNB1 a
rare genetic condition that means I have no peripheral vision,

no night vision,
and cannot detect movement the way others can.
Some years later I was told that I had 30% vision.

But until the time of my diagnosis,
no-one had noticed my sight was deficient.
I thought it was how everyone saw.

The team at Moorfields eye hospital,
led by an eminent professor were very excited.
I was just stunned in disbelief.

I couldn't believe other people saw things differently..
The excitement called for a celebration,
many peered into my eyes,
and champagne was promised for later,
but not for me.

They didn't have time to explain,
so I put the children back in the car
and drove back from London.

They could do nothing for my vision, so apart from going back to
help with their research they discharged me.

I finally stopped driving in 1993,
when I was 34,
and I finally had the courage to make an appointment at the local
eye hospital,
and could ask the question;
    "is it safe for me to drive?"
"Of course not. You've only got 30% vision"
was the reply,
no hesitation,
no question.
*The answer was **NO.***

"You can be registered as partially sighted or perhaps blind if that
helps?".

That was the end of my career as a visually impaired driver,
and although it was right to stop,
it was hard to give up.
Driving represented freedom,
and the "giving up" represented once again that I was
"useless".

I felt useless.

I couldn't drive the children here and there,
I couldn't drive.
Another thing lost

along with my dignity.

Most of the experiences shared so far are about the individual's personal response to losing sight and learning new ways of doing things, but, there is also the whole question of how other people's attitudes towards blindness and our difference affect our life experiences. My conversations with Tony reflected something of this:

Tony: a lot of visually impaired people are thought of
as mentally ill; aren't they?

Sue: or certainly not very bright!

I use that word carefully.
But I've been given almost a label.
Because, if you see somebody with a white stick...
although it's not it's not in ...
how shall I describe it...
like a lot of other illnesses,
you are thought of as mentally ill.
Even people in wheel chairs sometimes, aren't they?
I told you the one about;
many years ago,
I knew an old gentleman
who was an ex-manager of a department store,
who went blind,
and he used to go to the "Red Cross club".

He was asked all the time
if I was there talking to him..
"does he want" or his wife was asked,
"does he want a cakie?"
He was ..

Marginalised

Well a lot of disabled people,
even today feel that,
don't they?.....................

This is not being dramatic because I'm not..
just sometimes I have a feeling of ..
just walking out in the morning
and not coming back again...

Just walking out.

Well not coming back let's say.
Or thinking in my head ..

Of course I would never get round to do it...
I haven't got the ...
I've been emasculated.

So I'd stay here,
but I don't know whether any other people you talk to have told you
that sometimes they feel like this?...

Sue: Yes. Often

Just disappearing,
because they feel they've become a sort of
not so much a sort of burden,
but a non-entity.

Sue: So almost being invisible?

Yes. Yes.
Sometimes...

*Sue: and that kind of feeling "I can just walk out to nothingness
and..."*

Exactly.
You've hit the nail mostly on the head...
slightly..
probably a bit different
but you've hit the nail fairly firmly on the head...
That's because;
I'm not doing much.

I'm not doing much these days..
As I've told you about the reason I left the charity shop,
not because I didn't like the people who were there

I didn't want to be there as a fixture,

Sue: or as a token ...

Token...
token disabled person..
which I was more or less...

*Sue: But you think that since your sight has become worse
that feeling ...*

Has increased.
I mean I've got more used to not having sight,
but it's ...
difficult to come to terms with sometimes.
Although I do,
because,

I need to get through the day.

Simple tasks become difficult..
having to ask people to give me a hand
with washing and that...

Not washing me...
Washing clothes and things...
I mean I did my..

I tried to do some washing the other day,
but I put so much soap powder in;
because I didn't know how to gauge it
(and I've done that before as well by the way).
It came out with soap stuck all over it.

Sue: you said to me before that when you've been down in the past
perhaps you'd go out, but I'm wondering whether with less sight that
is more difficult to go out?

Yes.
I've got less inclination to go out..
and I should have inclination,
I don't want this place to become a prison,
but like now it's raining I shan't ...
no good going out unless ...
I don't know is there?
Is there?

Unless I go out ...

Get up and go out,
I'm apt to stay in.
Which makes it a very long day.

Luckily I know an elderly lady who I've known for 20 years, at least
twenty years..
getting on for 25 years,
who was a member of the Labour Party;
who I go and see because she's on her own,
she lost her husband some years ago,
and I used to visit him every week,
so that was something ..

Sue: A purpose for going?

A purpose,
I mean I go to Withywood University
but that's a university in name only it's not ...
He's a self styled eccentric!

I went to a concert;

something which I enjoyed better
was a concert at the church centre up the road the other day.

Sue: So those kind of events … you feel there's a purpose to going?

Yes it was folk music…
I went with some of the people up the road,
which was better,
because it was more …
it wasn't about a "so called" towering personality,
overruling just ordinary people.

*Sue: But that's a kind of attitude that you've talked about before,
one of "us and them" and "them and us"?*

Them and us,
yes. ..
and I'm not intimidated by these people by the way!
(laughter)

Sue: I can tell!

It's just that they frustrate me.
They're not their real self.
Which I know…
I put on a front.

Sue: We all put on a front!

But I don't put on an excessive front,
I just do it to survive.
You know.
If I told people I felt a bit miserable they wouldn't…
if they were miserable themselves
there wouldn't be much point would there?

*Sue: And if you said to somebody 'I just sometimes feel like walking
away…*

They would think …
they'd ring up the psychiatric unit (if there is one) ….
(laughter)

*Sue: It is something I've heard a lot from people,
because losing sight just makes everything…
it compounds life..*

Other problems

*Sue: that are difficult anyway,
it just makes them more difficult..
And if you've got more than one problem…*

which many people have by the way.
If you've got more than one difficulty,
it can..
as you know in talking to other people,
it can be very ...

it compounds as you say...
compounding...

Some people grieve for what they cannot see any more, others for what they cannot do, or for a life they lived prior to losing a sense, some feel frustrated and angry at societies inability to include their difference. For one man who contacted me following a presentation however losing sight was experienced by him as an opportunity. An opportunity for a new life.

George: At first I was in shock,
losing an eye,
being involved in an incident like that
It kind of brought me to my senses,
I had to start again,
Had to re-think my life – what was important.

It was like God gave me a kick up the bum and said:
"you have a new chance to do things differently"

Yes sometimes I get down and frustrated,
and it is difficult to admit to these feelings or my family think that I
am going back to my old ways (I was heavily into drink and drugs)
But, despite the pain I am embracing this new me – like a new friend
I have what so many people don't have,
the chance to start again as someone else.

The Etiquette of the sighted (Part Two)

The word "Blind" has different connotations to "visually impaired" "vision impaired" or "partially sighted". As Ferguson points out, fear of blindness and the linking this to "punishment" and "darkness" go back to biblical times where to "walk in darkness" had connotations of sin and despair, and to "walk in the light" meant to walk in God's presence (Ferguson 2001; Kinash 2005). As Kinash says, these images are not contradicted through journals such as the Journal for Visual Impairment and Blindness, and the British Journal for Visual Impairment, where medical models of blindness dominate, and the emphasis is on treatment and rehabilitation. She points out;

"Remarkably absent in antiquity and today is the experiential, the reflexive- the voice of the blind – particularly the voice of those who have re-claimed the idea of blindness" (Kinash 2005:37).

What I wonder does Kinash mean by the idea of blindness? Does she mean those who are totally blind, or people like me with a degree of blindness? And, how can we reclaim it I wonder? Perhaps she means that many of us play down, or try to ignore our visual impairment such that we "fit in" with what society expects of us.

Our language is littered with phrases implying sighted means "knowing" and blindness "ignorance". "Seeing is believing", and "I see what you mean" "out of sight out of mind" just three examples. So describing ourselves as "blind", especially if we have some residual vision, seems distinctly uncomfortable, and we are expected to conform to the etiquette of the sighted and live our lives in a sighted world without the sight, and live our lives with other people's perceptions of what that lack of sight or blindness may be like. If we challenge other people's opinions or as Kinash says, "re-claim the idea of blindness" as being ok, then we are labelled as, "defensive" or "failing to come to terms with things", by sighted people. How we re-claim blindness is also a matter of contention. One friend who is visually impaired teased me recently by saying, "you appear sighted, that doesn't help our cause. Can't you use your white cane a bit more?" Although it was said as a joke, there is a degree of truth, and makes me think that there is perhaps also an "etiquette of blindness", and if like me you do not fit in, then this can also be a very uncomfortable position.

Visually impaired people have been challenging communities' attitudes for decades. There were mass demonstrations of blind workers and sympathisers in London in 1920, 1933 and 1947 protesting against unemployment, low wages and poor working conditions (Humphries and Gordon 1992). Organisations supporting those who are blind and partially sighted have worked tirelessly within the disability rights movement whose ethos considers disabled people only disabled by societal attitudes and discriminatory practices. They have worked to promote social inclusion in both employment and social settings.

The largest organisation supporting people who are visually impaired is the USA's National Federation of the Blind, whose mission statement says:

"The mission of the National Federation of the Blind is to achieve widespread emotional acceptance and intellectual understanding that the real problem of blindness is not the loss of eyesight but the misconceptions and lack of information which exist". (NFB 2008)

Blindness within this context is not perceived as a disability, people who are blind are considered just ordinary people without sight. Neither is blindness seen as a culture (in the way that some within the Deaf community claim (Jones and Bunton 2008)) the focus is very much on integration within society, a society which accepts "sighted" as normal.

RNIB is the UK's biggest organisation which espouses to "support blind and partially sighted people". Their mission statement says that it aims:

> "To challenge blindness by empowering people who are blind or partially sighted, removing the barriers they face and helping to prevent blindness" (RNIB 2008).

Again the emphasis is on integration within society, and "preventing blindness" the latter being a value statement inferring that sight is better than blind!

To reiterate, the social model has encouraged many positive changes in the environment we live in such as: more accessible buildings and transport systems, access to work schemes which provide accessible technology and support for disabled employees, documents and books being available in different reading formats. These have all made life easier for those of us with limited vision, but, they have often been offered in such a way as to encourage visually impaired people to make light of their sensory loss, and to live life within the sighted paradigms, such that they fit in. For example recently in conversation with a social services rehabilitation officer I was told, "we have to train people to think positively about the sight they have, and how they can fit into society again so they can feel productive and useful, this will probably mean they have to learn not to talk about the things they find difficult, otherwise they will be excluded."

This way of thinking has had many positive outcomes, people with visual impairments have succeeded in many areas of life, but, I consider that it has sometimes disabled people "emotionally", not giving them space to voice their thoughts and feelings about the experience of losing sight, and their experience of living with a visual impairment. Societal beliefs about blindness therefore remain unchanged, apart from recognising the need to have accessible information, and this means in practice that often as a blind person, to get on, one has to collude and make light of sensory loss and work so much harder to get to the same position within employment, social or political settings.

To give an example of this, one young woman on a graduate training scheme that I met with last year talked of how she was required by her employer to present "power-point spread sheets", which were not accessible to her, (and not compatible with her computer text reader) at team meetings. She unlike her sighted colleagues, had to memorise every figure contained in the spread-sheet, and when her employer was challenged about this said: "The government has provided you with specialist equipment. Now you have to do things in the same way as everyone else. Why should you have special privileges? We consider you to be **just the same** as everyone else, and you **should be grateful** that we don't discriminate".

In my opinion equal opportunities should be about inclusive practices, not treating everyone the same, and also about giving space for people to say how they feel, whether that is positive, or negative, or perhaps ambivalent.

I was very interested in how people who had lived with a visual impairment for a long time would respond to the stories about recent sight loss. Following a conference where I presented stories from Andy and Sarah[2] I met Will who was also a counsellor and lived in Aukland New Zealand. Will describes himself as "a successful blind man" he has RP and over the years has gradually lost sight. He comments that despite living with a visual impairment most of his life he still fears losing more vision. He sent me this poem he had recently written:

Will:
The dark has come again
I'm so afraid
of blackness overwhelming me.
Waking in the night
I can't tell;
have I lost the last remnants of sight?
I lay motionless.
Voiceless.
So afraid.

My wife sleeps beside me unaware.
Sweat rolls down my face,
I cannot bear another moment of not knowing.
I get out of bed and go to the washroom
I switch the light on.
And sit silently weeping.
A little light remains,
But for how long?
I am to those around me a successful blind man
with a career and a wife.

---

[2] "Knitting in the Dark: having conversations about living with a visual impairment" was presented at the International Conference of Narrative Therapy and Community Work in Norway in 2008

I tell myself that blindness does not matter
But deep inside my soul states:
I hate being fucking blind.
I am afraid of the dark

Patrick emails me and we start a conversation:

Hi Sue,
When I first read some of your stories about the experience of losing sight I felt really angry. It felt like everything I had worked so hard for over the years had crumbled away. The story I have always told of myself as being well adjusted, happy, successful, a blind man who did not mind being blind felt under threat. I wept when I read Andy and Sarah's story and then felt really angry with them, with you. My world felt as if perhaps it was just a façade that I put up to hide how I felt about blindness about being different. I'm not sure I really know what blindness is. I can't remember seeing, so I don't know what that means either. I do know that being labelled blind by others has been tough, and some people can do things because of a sense they have and I am without. All my life I have had to fight for a place for myself in society. At work, at home. I have fought to maintain the image of someone successful, someone who is "different" rather than blind. I have always been afraid that if I ever say anything negative about being blind this will be interpreted as "poor Patrick" and I will be seen as a victim and pitied, and I couldn't bear that. I always avoid people who have just been diagnosed with sight loss, their grief seems to tell me that my life experience is not ok, that I shouldn't feel happy. This was certainly something that was hammered home at school. We were only seen as successful blind students if we were positive and rose to the challenge – rather like the saintly Helen Keller[3]. It is also I think about perhaps the suspicion that I have been kidding myself that not having sight is ok. Perhaps I need to allow myself to feel the negatives as well as the positives. What do you think?

> Dear Patrick,
> I'm not sure I've got any simple answers. I think the whole of our lives is about positive and negative experiences, and perhaps we need to acknowledge both the positives and the negatives. As you know my sight has always been the same. I haven't "lost" sight, but I still feel at times angry, sad – loss of what could have been if only I had better sight. I feel angry that I was seen as "useless" rather than visually impaired. To think of visual impairment as a "personal tragedy to be overcome"

---

[3] Kleege writes "Many disabled people think you (Helen Keller) did our cause a lot of harm. Your life story inscribes the idea that disability is a personal tragedy to be overcome through an individual's fortitude and pluck, rather than a set of cultural practices and assumptions, affecting many individuals that could be changed through collective action" (Kleege 2006:1)

makes me feel quite nauseous as I don't feel in the slightest "tragic" but not to be able to acknowledge the frustrations and feelings (both bad and good) about how being visually impaired impacts on my life experiences would limit my ability to be me and put a label on what being visually impaired means. Does this make any sense or am I just rambling?

Hi Sue,
I think you are right. I know that I have huge feelings of rage, of sadness that I have never expressed, and they don't take away from my ability to be successful and happy, but there is always the fear that if I do express them I am letting down the "blind community" who gain strength through their solidarity that being blind is ok. But this leaves people who are losing sight with no community to support them. They are rejected by the blind community for feeling that being blind is not ok and also rejected by the sighted community as being "less than" sighted.

Mike is a colleague and friend, and also engaged in doctoral research exploring "the theology of disability" with the University of Aberdeen, so I had no hesitation in sharing the stories from my research with him, initially these were the stories from Andy and Sarah and this is the response I received:

Dear Sue,

[4]Knitting In the Dark Reflection
It's a strange experience listening to the deep experiences of sight loss in their rawest state. I started reading 'Knitting In The Dark' at my desk at 4.18 pm - it was kind of an act of defiance, probably not something that should have been at the top of my list of things to do, but it had been a frustrating day - part of a frustrating week - and I wanted to read it, so why not.

It's still a new experience for me - metaphorically picking up something to read and not being able to put it down. Filled with anger and amazement, joy and sadness I race through 23 pages of the paper - empathetic one second, and horrified the next. I had to stop reading, the trains won't wait for me.

Left the building, plunged into the indistinct greyness of twilight - if I was walking on the sky, I'd be able to see where I was going. Tapped along the pavement, got to the crossing - a mother and child get to the crossing and press the button before me, and tell me so - the same thing happens at the island - I explain that I want to stand by the box so that I can feel the rotating cone on the bottom - they

---

[4] This email and the following one from Will was originally published as part of an article in TSI-Theory in action see Dale 2008b and reproduced here with permission.

seem interested. I feel a sense of joy that my difference has provoked such a fleeting yet warm encounter that they have probably forgotten - or have they?

Over the bridge and up the long road towards Temple Meads, passing by the huge shadowy trees - I think I can see them, but I'm not sure about the ones I can't see. I know its silly, but I still get excited about going on trains - yes, at the age of 37, I still get excited - even at just a 6 minute journey. I guess its partly for the reasons that most of us like trains if we're honest - but for me its more than that. There is a sense of equality - we all have the same level of control, we are all equally unable to burst into the cab and take control of the destiny of the train.

I walk reflecting on the paper - I feel so happy that people have been given the opportunity to share their stories in such a graphic way - I feel angry? Hurt? I don't know... how can a life experience that I find so beautiful, such a gift, be so abhorrent to others - my words not theirs. Then I think... is my experience beautiful, or is it just the conditioning of my unwavering loyalty to the social understanding (I've given up the word model at least) of Disability. Yes, it is a beautiful gift and I'm damn well going to prove it on the rest of my journey.

I walk further, past the bus stop and the yellow bridge - I can't see that it's yellow anymore in this light - but that doesn't take away from its yellowness. There's a road sign coming up somewhere - two vertical poles in the middle of the pavement - it's a road sign for cars, why can't they put it in the road then - after all car drivers by definition can see, they could drive round it - I guess my way round it - what justice is there in that? The sign approaches - I see it silhouetted against the grey sky - feeling quietly pleased with my powers of observation.

I don't like walking this route in the dark or almost dark, and yet the sense of achievement once I've completed it is worth it - is that how we're supposed to feel - I don't care, navigating a mile of pavements, trees, sign posts, crossings, traffic etc etc. blooming well is (sorry, but I don't swear - why I am I apologising)?

Complicated crossing coming up, recently fitted tactile cones - I've been on at them about that for years - wonder if I made any difference, probably not! Strange angle to cross at, will I get it right - almost - a bit of adjustment required - always know that I'm in the right place when I get blinded by the headlights of the cars on the other side of the roundabout. Cross over the middle of the roundabout, over the second road and approach the third - tactile cone rotates - I wonder if they did take any notice of me - start crossing, I become aware of a car parked over the crossing - I tap it with my stick anyway - is that naughty? Just trying to make a point...

I always seem to want to know the time at this point, to see how much time I've got - like I can run for it to make up the lost minutes! Loads of time. Only one little road to cross and I'm on the station approach - airport bus goes by - I can tell it's the airport bus because it has bright illuminated signs on the front and side and looks bigger than a normal bus - whatever a normal bus is. I love flying - can't believe it after failing to turn up for a flight two years ago because I was so scared. I love being treated like a human being at the airport - being offered assistance instead of grabbed - being made to feel special - not in a patronising way, just in a way that we should all be made to feel special sometimes. I love the sensations - take off, landing - seeing the clouds, the sun on otherwise gloomy days - flying to Glasgow in two days. It's a pity it will be dark, never mind - still looking forward to it - I still love adventures. Does God mind me flying? I wonder, its not very good for my green credentials. Perhaps I'm allowed - feels a bit like asking for compensation - that seems to imply that my living with a visual impairment needs compensating for - not really, but surely if there are some visual experiences that I can't have, then I'm entitled to make the most of others.

I've been using this station for more than 20 years, still get in a bit of a pickle with the ticket windows - can see some people standing at windows - I'll just try to replace them when one moves, not sure if anyone else is waiting. Exchange light hearted conversation with the ticket seller - said that I'd heard about the refurbished trains on the news - he said that he doesn't trust the news! I tried to keep positive. I ask for a platform number - he's really friendly, it makes such a difference. Make my way onto the platform - there's a train in - I head for the lights which I think illuminate the vestibule - they do - I ask the space if this is the train to Keynsham - there is an affirming voice in the space and I climb aboard. A few of us stand and I exchange pleasantries about the over-crowding. I love trains, so glad I don't have the choice of whether to drive or not. Taxi company call, my driver will be late at the station - so would I as the train progressed slowly. Got of the train after about 10 or 12 minutes - its strange, people can be so helpful and yet so often at Keynsham no one offers assistance. At that moment a woman asks if I need a hand - I take her arm - I love that intimate encounter with strangers - the privilege of walking as one for a few moments on our shared journey of life. Seconds later the taxi pulls up and I am greeted by the driver. We share the events of our days together for the 9 minute journey, such a nice guy.

Not an easy journey I know - but if I was fully sighted it wouldn't be the same, I may not have even caught the train or climbed into a taxi - I certainly wouldn't have had the innocently intimate encounters with strangers that I have so often. I don't want to see any less, of course not. But neither can I imagine seeing everything - it just wouldn't be me, I'd turn into someone else - just like Molly Sweeney. I know I shouldn't be hurt, but sometimes I feel it when what I think of such a beautiful gift is so painful to others. Perhaps even my thought of partial sight as a gift is hurtful to them too. Of

course, life is tough, more difficult, physically tiring, sometimes
logistically complicated - but I don't think I want to swap it - I am
who I am - I am who God made me, and that's good enough for me'
(Dale 2008b).

Will follows up his poem with an email:

Hi Sue
I have never been allowed to say "this isn't alright"
or,
"I hate being fucking blind"
You have given me permission to   say that...
It is hard to put into words how that affects me...
How much I have needed to say:
I hate being blind.
I hate that I cannot see.
That there is this whole part of life which I miss out on.
That everything – even with the right equipment
takes twice as long.
Sue, you mentioned that one of your client's responses to you telling
him of coming to the conference was,
"if they want to   know what blindness is like,
just give them a 6 inch nail and a hammer
and ask them to drive it through their foot".

Blindness is bloody and painful.
I think on the whole I "accept" my blindness,
and I live a satisfying life
but why can't I be allowed to grieve, shout, sob about it.
Why do I have to be grateful all the time about what I can do?
(Dale 2008b).

CHAPTER THREE

CHANGING RELATIONSHIPS

This chapter focuses on how the dynamics of personal relationships change with loss of sight and how this is experienced by both those losing the sight and also the effects on families and friends. It also includes part three of commentary "the etiquette of the sighted". May comments:

> May: I've always been the strong one
> and looked after him.
> You know,
> cooking and fussing.
> Now I am blind the tables are turned,
> and I don't like it.
> I don't like it at all,
> and neither does he!
> It is like this malevolent person is coming between us.
> Blindness.
> Mr. B!

May and her husband had requested to meet with me following May's diagnosis of age related macular degeneration (AMD) which had resulted in May losing most of her central vision and her being registered as seriously sight impaired (blind). They both considered that "blindness" was affecting May's confidence, making her depressed and was "coming between them". May was unsure about counselling thinking that "all that touchy feely stuff isn't really for me. We were always told 'stiff upper lip' and got on with it". You will hear more of my work with May and Peter in later chapters, but wanted to include May's words here as they were sentiments common for many of the people consulting me who were affected by recent sight loss. Loss of sight seemed in some way to come between people. Annie talks to me about her experiences:

> Annie: The hardest thing is not being able to see people's faces
> when they talk to me,
> it just makes it so hard to feel close to them.
> I was trying to support a friend of mine who had some bad news,
> she sat on the sofa,
> I sat beside her,
> but there was this infuriating blankness between us.
> I tried to say the right things,

but I just felt so out of touch with her.

It is hard with (name) and the children as well.
I can't be who I used to be for them all,
I am still really close to my daughter,
but my husband finds it very difficult.
He won't talk about it with me
I know he worries,
his way is to pretend it is not happening.
That means that at times he expects me to do things I can't possibly do now,
and that leaves me feeling like a failure!

Adam who was diagnosed with RP as a child talks with me about relationships too with regard to his degenerative condition:

Adam: As regard my condition...
It is degenerative,
and it has slowly deteriorated over the 33 years;
and I think degenerative conditions
are just so ...so difficult.

I'm not saying they're more difficult
than somebody that loses all their vision overnight,
but the consistency of that
It is obviously a huge loss,
and a huge thing to get used to,
but it is consistent.

I think one of the difficult things I find,
and still do,
is...
being so grateful for the vision that I have,
and yet, having
such frustration,
and such resentment
and such loss.

It's such a difficult tension to hold
because
you ...

in some ways you want to commit visual suicide;
because you know it is happening
and yet there is another side of me
that is so blessed
and so grateful,
and so appreciative for the vision I do have,
which is very little now,
but....
I'm still wired up

very, very visually,
so I still operate thinking in that way,
so I find it very difficult
at times.
I think the other problem I find,
and I constantly find with
deterioration or degenerative issues
is the fact that if you are,
or if you have learnt to become a good communicator,
and you do care about others around you,
and you do communicate where you are,
how you're feeling,
what you can see
and what you can't see,
then if you are really good at communicating, what you communicate today
will be different in three or four weeks,
or 5 months time.
And I'm starting to realise that the better my communication,
the more mistrust I can breed in some relationships;
because people don't realise, that they don't have your experience of loss
and transition,
and they don't realise that things can change.
And they say,
"well I thought you could see that.
You told me that you could see that,
and now you're telling me you can't".

And it is really difficult,
and I think that it's so hard to actually be,
"who you are in that moment"
as a visually impaired person,
because; you're always considering
the impact of being authentic in a relationship,
because it is very difficult to be authentic
because,
how can you verbalise how beautiful a yellow daffodil looks over there;
when you've just told them that
"you can't do something because of lack of vision",
and demanded their support.

It's really difficult.

Sue: So it changes the dynamic of the relationship?

Yes it does,
I think it compromises...
I do feel that my visual impairment
compromises my ability to be authentic in a relationship,
and it's a real challenge to be truly authentic

and true to yourself in company.

Whilst I appreciate that ….
I think there's something very mysterious about sight loss.
I think a lot of people that spend time with me they don't actually
use the word …
They don't articulate it like that,
but I know that they find me very mysterious,
they don't know what I can see,
they don't know when I can see,
they don't know what I'm processing,
how much of an experience am I sharing?
and it's very, very mysterious,
and mystery quite often leads to fantasy,
and people..
people operate so very differently around me
it's unbelievable.

Sue: What… compared to other people?

Yes I think so.
Yes. I feel they do.

Sue: Certainly I think I identify with that
because when ..
I can fake it as being sighted most of the time,
and have done it most of my life.

It changes the dynamic ..
in the moment
I think,
when I tell people what I can see,
and what I can't see, it …
I agree, it does change the dynamic.

I think the thing which I am possibly struggling with the most at the
moment
and … this is linked into
identity
and masculinity
is …

primarily,
to do with being in relationship with other people in the world,
I think that being ….
I cope
better
if I exclude myself,
and operate almost in an adaptive isolating environment,
though that is not the way I want to live my life..

Sue: so I mean…

how do you do that?

Well I don't know
(laughter)
all I know that is;
what I'm currently trying to do
is include myself in as many aspects of human experience
as I can,
and it's really difficult.

It is very, very difficult....
and I know that probably that dynamic is not exclusive
to somebody with sight loss,
because,
it is difficult to be in relationship with the world,
and others
isn't it?

But
I think there's something about sight loss
that makes it
very, very difficult.

Michael emails me after he has listened to Adam's story having borrowed my audio-thesis from the university library:

Hi Sue,
One of the things that really struck me when I listened to Adam's story was this whole question of how blindness had affected my ability to relate to others, my work colleagues, people I pass in the street, my friends and family, and even the relationship I had with my now ex-wife.

As my condition got worse people who at the beginning had been very supportive and shocked when I told them seemed to lose patience with the things I now couldn't do. Where I used to go down the pub with the lads and play darts they no longer invited me. People, even those who knew I had a sight problem would often say things like "why did you ignore me when we were walking through town yesterday?" When I was able to see something, because the lighting was ok or I had caught sight of it out of the corner of my eye people would say things like "I thought you couldn't see? You saw that as well as I did". I felt a fraud, and stopped telling people when I could see things, somehow it was easier if they assumed that I couldn't see at all, but even that didn't work, because I began to feel alienated. People just didn't want to talk to me any more.

I had been married for 13 years when I was diagnosed, my wife (name) was very supportive, has always been supportive, but it has changed things between us. In fact we are now permanently separated, I'm not sure that is totally down to the sight loss, but it was a contributing factor, of that I am sure.

From her perspective I guess it is very hard when the man you are married to and has always been the bread winner and the "man of the house" becomes dependant on you for everything from being transported to cutting your toenails. I couldn't tell whether she had just had her hair done, was in a really sexy dress or whether she was in her old jeans. It sounds as if these are really small things, and I guess on their own they are, but they niggle between you and eventually she found someone who wasn't so dependent on her.

Matt also emails me following a conversation at a conference where I had been presenting stories about the emotional impact of diagnosis and registration:

Hi Sue,
You asked me "what kinds of things have changed?" for me since being registered as blind.

Well I suppose one of the biggies is my relationship with my partner and children.

It went from me being the one who went out to work, provided the main income, the one who only saw the kids in the evenings at weekends, who always had a company car and all the perks to me being at home, on benefits (my partner now works full time) seeing the kids after school and having to travel by bus everywhere, and being depressed most of the time. We met and made commitments to each other when I was a totally different person, and I think it is just as hard for her as it is for me. She didn't ask for any of this to happen, and I feel guilty that she is having to put up with it. We don't row, but somehow we are not as close as we used to be, and I am scared sometimes that she might find someone else with less problems.

It has been good to see more of the kids – although to start with it was tricky because again I was different to the Dad they used to have.

The etiquette of the sighted (Part Three)

It seems very difficult sometimes for the sighted and the visually impaired to communicate effectively, partly I consider, because the sighted do not necessarily think much about their sight, and take for granted that "seeing is normal" and blindness is definitely "not normal". When we as visually impaired people assume an attitude of playing down our blindness and the effect it has on our lives and comply with these sighted assumptions about life, this can, in the short term, enable us to fit in, and feel accepted, and in some senses we have an easier life, but it can also leave us feeling not listened to and without a voice.

Davis in 1961 pointed out that during social interactions between able bodied, and disabled people difference was often dissipated by the able bodied with a leading comment such as,

"I don't think of you as disabled" – so unthinkingly confirming the latter's tragic fate. The 'well adjusted' disabled person is someone who lives up to non-disabled people's expectations as brave, cheerful and grateful when being helped" (cited in Barnes and Mercer 2003:7).

As Dennis so aptly says "we have to be so grateful all the time, grateful for help that we don't want to have to ask for". Scott also identified that people who were blind were rewarded for assimilating the beliefs of the experts, and rehabilitation teams (Scott 1969). There is as Kinash states a culture of compliance, "compliance not only with societal rules and regulations but with normality" (Kinash 2005:33).

The stories from Knitting in the Dark, and indeed the stories emerging from by doctoral project and this book do not fit in with this culture of compliance, they are often experienced as uncomfortable and disturbing by those who are sighted. An ophthalmologist at a recent conference said to me "I found these stories very difficult to hear. I have always thought of sight loss as a medical disorder, to think of it in a non-medical way is deeply disturbing, but essential if I am to help people more effectively". Stories, however, often evoke stories (Speedy 2008) and some people who are visually impaired have found the stories liberating in that it has given them permission to voice their thoughts and feelings, whatever those may be. Some have spoken about their positive experiences of being blind, which cut across the presumptions that blindness is always tragic, and others have spoken about how difficult being blind can be.

Fergusson (2001) and Kinash (2005) go on to illuminate the tension between the needs of people who are visually impaired and the attitudes and services provided by the professionals paid to support them, "emerging through the absence of opportunity for the blind to voice their opinions or take a functional role in the formation of policy and procedure" (Kinash 2005:27). If there is an attitude of "compliance" then it is very difficult for blind or partially sighted people to have a voice. And when we do take on a role in the formation of policy and procedure and speak against the grain, so to speak, we are often judged by our visual acuity rather than our ability. On a personal note, even working for a leading charity supporting people who are blind or partially sighted, and coming into post with an excellent C.V. and references I was told by a manager when leaving, "I am really surprised at how well you have done. I was really worried when you said that you were visually impaired, that you wouldn't be able to do the job". He was not being unkind, just truthful, and demonstrated to me why so many of us "play down" or minimise the effect our lack of vision has on our life. But doing this I believe has a personal cost, it means denying part of who we are, and feelings of not fully accepted as who we are by the people we are with.

Being the "Other Half"

Over the last few years Dennis and I have talked about many aspects of visual impairment including what it must be like to be the "other half" or the partner of someone who like ourselves has a visual impairment.

Dennis: Of course there's one position that you and I
and people with vision problems like ourselves
haven't been in;
Being the other half
of somebody that's visually impaired.

Sue: I think that's huge as well.
The impact on partners,
hopefully when people have a very good relationship
they ..
we all adapt to the needs of our partners don't we?

We do, but....
With the onset of visual impairment in one partner,
there is an inevitable shift within their relationship
that might be not wanted,
or found difficult to deal with
and is about that business of
tasks changing,
and for me the obvious one is
I had to stop driving
so wherever we go now my wife's got to drive.
So when she gets fed up driving,
how does that affect me?

It makes me just think '***why can't I do it?***'

Sue: I can identify with that.
To see that other partner tired driving.
And you think "***why can't I do this***?"
For me it's anger that sets in I think..

It is.
But the problem is,
because she's tired,
and I'm angry

that is a recipe for disaster.

Because we could end up taking it out on each other
for the completely wrong reasons.
Yet you're available
(laughter)
and you're there.
Just the two of you.

As I say that's just driving..
there's numerous other things
just thinking of one or two examples here ..

there are just so many.

Well,
something as simple as washing up.
I guess I could be accused of being a little bit of a cheat here,
and perhaps doing it on purpose
but I don't.
    I don't mind helping with the dishes,
but (name deleted) has said to me,
"let me do them because if you do them
I'm only going to have to do them again
because you miss bits".

Sue: But that reinforces the …

Yes. **It does**
absolutely,
and when we cut the lawn, I've got a big lawn,
I do all the main middle bit,
but she'll do the edges,
because she's worried I'm going to chop the flowers down,
because I just miss the lawn,
my judgment is poor.

But it just goes on and on doesn't it.
You can just think of so many...
I certainly could.

Talking to you today
I've really reinforced one of the decisions I've made.
It's like I wish the opportunity would present itself
to see if I actually have got the courage to do it.

But the next time somebody says to me
"I thought you were blind?"
and in a kind of
jokey, mocking, teasing way
which is not really meant to be hurtful
    (they don't realise how I feel about that comment)

I am actually going to say,
"has it ever occurred to you,
or do you ever think
how that might make me feel
when you say that".

I really am going work very hard
and hope I have the courage to say that.

Sue: That will be very interesting to see what kind of reaction you get to that!

And I'm a dreadful one for predicting,
but I would predict
that what they might say is
"I was only kidding,
I was only messing around,
don't be so sensitive".

So in other words you get it straight back.

So how would I respond to that?
or would I just accept that.
Knowing me, I would think that in accepting
 that I'm acknowledging that they're right
that I'm too sensitive,
so I've lost the initiative.
And I don't want to lose the initiative.

So maybe I need to think about that a little bit more
in case somebody does say to me,
"I was only kidding you know"
I'll say to them,
"well you saying I'm a bit sensitive
actually,
yes you're right, I am a bit sensitive,
and that's why I don't …
share your joke.
I don't actually share your joke"

Sue: it's funny that I can laugh about myself
doing strange things
like ..
walking into the gents the other week ..
very helpfully instead of putting the normal signs up
they'd painted the one door pale blue and the other pale pink.
To me they both looked a nice shade of grey (Laughter).
I picked one and it was the gents..
there was a man standing at the urinals.
"Oh so very sorry"…
I can laugh about it but if anybody else says,
"Oh God! your eyesight's terrible ..

you went through the wrong door…"
and made it as a joke
it would be really painful.
So there's something for me about
I can do it,
the laughing about me,
but I don't want other people to do it.

No. That's right.
That's right.

Sue: I've had many interesting experiences in the gents!

Do you want to talk about it now?

Sue: (Laughter) …
"It's a good job I can't see very well" is usually my comment!

Will emails me in response to Mike's reflection on knitting in the dark (see chapter two):

Hi Sue,
I am delighted that you want to include my story in your writing. I have read through these new stories, and they have moved me to tears yet again!

I think that I can understand a bit about what Mike is saying. Being accepted by others has been huge for me too. There all my life. I'm never just Will, but often "the guy who is blind". It is ok for me and liberating to say "I hate being blind". But it is not ok for others to assume they know how I do, or should feel. I am not just blind, I am a dad, a poet, a lover, a cook, a therapist and I live my life ensuring that these stories are more important than "blind". I have realised however that for me to move to any place where I can accept blindness as a "gift" and part of who I am, I have to allow myself to feel the negative unexpressed feelings which contaminate these other parts of me. Your stories have shown me hope.

Journal October 11th 2008

Following the end of my career as a visually impaired driver, I started on a new career; the visually impaired passenger and map-reader.

The peculiarities of my vision mean that: I can see the centre of the map quite well so, if I know where we are in relation to the map, and where we are going is in the centre of the map, I can usually say helpfully, "take the next left", or "take the next right". I can even mostly know the number of the road we are on and the one we are aiming for. Providing that there is no ambiguity, my map reading is successful.

Where it falls apart however, and sometimes causes marital strife, is when I need to be able to see the road-signs and the points of reference that are actually beside the road. However hard I try, I can never see them in time. by the time I have focussed on a particular sign, it has gone, and another has passed away that I didn't see at all!

We now I hasten to say have Emily, who on the whole has taken the stress out of navigating. Her satellites do not require me to "see" things. She speaks calmly, doesn't mind being shouted at, and is eminently more up to the task than me. She is of course our sat-nav system.

She did fail us however earlier this year when we were trying to circumnavigate Dijon…

She and I definitely had different ideas on the best way forward, and she wanted to take our rather large 3 meter high camper van through very small back lanes and tunnels. Help!

We certainly needed the aperitif at the end of that day!

CHAPTER FOUR

EMPLOYMENT, STUDY AND BENEFITS

This chapter explores the experience of changing patterns in employment, study and what living on benefits is like. It includes part four of the commentary "the etiquette of the sighted".

Journal 10 October 2008

*I was invited today to a meeting just outside Llanidloes. "Would you like to come? It should only last a couple of hours!" Yes. I would like to go. Attending would be really interesting, Llanidloes is only about 20 miles away, but, unfortunately, **not on a bus route** from here.*

I looked up the services. It would take me 3 changes of bus, and over 4 hours (if they all run on time!) and I couldn't get there until after the meeting was over. A taxi? Well the cost would probably be about £40 each way and also a charge for waiting time.

*Do they want me to go **that much? Do I want to go that much?***

*Years ago I would have said nothing, I would have been worried that if I said, "I am going to find it difficult to get there" that they would reject me. I would have either begged a lift, or forked out for the taxi, and said nothing, done anything so that others wouldn't perceive me as weak, **or useless..***

I was afraid always of rejection, of being left out, losing my job, unemployable.

*Now I speak my mind. "As I don't drive (they know I'm partially sighted) and Llanidloes is not on a bus route from here I can only come if you supply a taxi!" "Oh yes. I forgot that you don't drive, it's **such** a nuisance, **I was** really relying on your input!"*

Several of the contributors to this book have cited their experience of education, both within special schools and within mainstream education as being important factors in how they view their visual impairment and also themselves. So the chapter starts with conversations about schooling. For those interested specifically in education and visual impairment see French, Swain et al (French et al. 2006) who used an oral history project to collect stories from

people who were visually impaired on their experiences of
education. The chapter then moves to employment issues adult
education and the effect of the benefit system.

Adam like myself went to a mainstream school, and when we met
to talk about his experience of living with a visual impairment this is
what he said:

Adam: As you know I have Retinitis Pigmentosa
and had rather a misunderstood childhood,
because I wasn't diagnosed until I was 9/10 years old,
and ...
I would say suffered quite a bit because of that.
Very misunderstood,
punished for things,
excluded from things,
and included when it was dangerous for me;
in all sorts of different things.
Quite a difficult time.

Sue: So was that because ...
nobody knew that your vision was ...

Nobody knew,
although mum and dad did suspect
and a couple of times they took me to the doctor
and I did even go to the hospital;
but they did not pick it up.
They just said,
"he's frightened of the dark, give him a kick up the bum".
So that's what mum and dad did
because they were listening to the professionals.

So...
however the turning point for me
was when I was in a stage production at school,
and I knew I couldn't cope with acting,
but I didn't understand enough about my condition
to say no to being a stage hand,
and so I agreed to not act.

But I agreed to help out
when the lights went down to remove all the furniture (laughter)
and I fell off in front of 4-500 people in the middle of the stage.
And that was...
that was it.
So,
at that point it completely changed my life...
When I was diagnosed,
I think it also changed my parents' life;

I managed to get through mainstream school
and got some GCSE's,
and had a really difficult teenage period really,
because everyone else was out doing things
and I was in.

I couldn't go out because it was dark,
and …
I was taught long cane in the last couple of years of my mainstream
education and …
didn't really understand why I was learning it,
but I was just being a good boy really
and kind of going along with it,
not realising that I would really need to use it one day,
and it was valuable.
And I was…
the worst,
and the only
visually impaired person in mainstream education,
up 'till 16.

I was registered blind at 15
and then,
I went from being the worst and only visually impaired person in this
school
to being one of the best visual people in a blind institution at 16.
So the change of psychology was just huge for me.

Sue: So what was it like going through mainstream …
was that a good decision do you think?

I was never offered anything different,
I mean nowadays
there's a lot more inclusion,
and a lot more support,
but I mean there was none of that then,
so I was just bumbling through
and I can't…
I don't know how I dealt with it,
looking back.
I just don't know how I dealt with it.
I was knocking over conical flasks of hydrochloric acid in the science
laboratory,
all over people's legs,
and all sorts of awful things happened,
but nobody removed me from the dynamic,
or supported me,
it was just …

Sue: You just got on with it

Yes.

I think the best thing that happened
was the P.E. teacher decided to buy a white cricket ball,
(laughter)
but he still continued to put me in the cricket nets.

And that is **awful** because ....
there's **nowhere to run** or hide
or anything...
in a cricket net...
knowing a ball is coming at you.

But he felt like he'd made an effort obviously...

Going to
a college for the blind at 16 years old was a huge change.
Massive transition,
and it was very liberating for me to be with other people that
obviously shared similar experiences.

It was liberating for me to separate myself from a family that
couldn't support me
because they found it so difficult..

Sue: and was that because of the practicalities,
or was that more about the...

It was emotional.
Emotional.
They just couldn't go there,
and didn't,
and not because they didn't care,
they just didn't,
they couldn't cope with it.
They are lovely people,
but they couldn't do it,
and still can't.
Despite the way I live my life,
which I think you know,
is very full and rich.

Several people responded to Adams Account. Ann emailed me
saying:

Hi Sue,
Sorry that it's taken such a long time to get back to you. Here's my
thoughts/response - I'm happy for you to use them but would be
grateful if you could keep them anonymous.

My first response, particularly to Adam's story was to get quite upset
- I'm going through a difficult time at the moment and it reminded
me so much of my own childhood. I'm in my mid 40's now and only

just realizing that I still have to come to terms with being visually impaired.

I'm lucky in that my condition has not and hopefully will not change - but I have very poor sight and am registered blind, I can however "pass" for sighted as I can read small print if I hold it close and so spent a lot of my childhood and early adult life pretending I could see. I mostly wasn't conscious of this but realise now that that's what I was doing.

Like Adam school was a nightmare, I still shudder when I hear the word "rounders" - images of standing on a wet, soggy common in south London with an entire class shouting at me to "catch it!" with me looking up and thinking "catch what?!". Always getting picked last for teams, never being asked out by boys and getting teased because of my funny eyes and a constant struggle to maintain this façade that I was normal and like everyone else. My way of dealing with it was to find ways round things e.g. copying friend's notes because I couldn't see the blackboard and waiting until the bus was right up to the stop before stepping forward to get on it.

Being visually impaired, or disabled in anyway is actually quite an effort – it means everyday we have to think of ways around things or plan things differently. And you can't get away from the fact that society does judge us, whether we like it or not!

Anna also emails me in response to listening to Adam's story picking up on the experience of education.

Hi Sue,
When I listened to Adam on the CD I found myself in tears – not for him, he sounds as if he is a really well adjusted person, but tears for me. Remembering my own school days and how difficult it was for me. I too was the only visually impaired person in our school. I had some vision but not enough to read the board, or to read normal size text. I did have a couple of hours a week one to one with a lady called Mrs Divine, who came in to help photocopy text books into large print and sometimes she would help me with spelling and maths. I feel I lost large chunks of school though because often I did not know what was going on, and some of the teachers were not able to give me the time I needed. There was also the bullying. I was an easy target and I looked different.

I hated school, especially sports. Adam's description of his sports teacher buying a white ball and thinking he had done all he could was so true to form. Yes a white ball is better than a grey one, but if you cannot see things moving then it still hurts!

I always wished that I could have gone to school somewhere where there were other blind people, I think it would have helped me to feel "part of something" rather than excluded.

My conversations with Mike take a different turn. He attended a residential school specifically for children who were visually impaired:

> Mike: I suppose I'd always seen my visual impairment
> in a fairly negative light.
> I think, a lot of my experience, in life,
> when I was at school
> was negative.
>
> I've got a reasonable amount of residual vision,
> but, even then I tended to be at the
> lower end of the spectrum.
> So it was always an object of
> teasing….
>
> Just always made to feel inferior to other people,
> because, I couldn't play football and all that sort of thing.
> I suppose it was also the reason why I was separated from my family;
> because I had to go away to school from the age of 5.
>
> So I think for a lot of my life it was a very negative thing.
>
> *Sue: There's a huge peer pressure thing?*
> *And if you stand outside that it's quite a painful place to be?*
>
> I think yes,
> because this was;
> other children with a visual impairment,
> and I think that this can almost be worse.
> (laughter)
>
> Academically, I suppose it did me well,
> but I think I lost a huge amount of confidence,
> I mean going away at 5 you don't have a lot of chance to build it!
>
> *Sue: It must have been very hard going away at 5..*
>
> Being separate from my family
> was hard,
> probably harder for my family..
>
> But something that has just occurred to me actually;
> that..
> when you go into that kind of environment,
> you're having to work very hard
> at feeling loved.
>
> *Sue: Because in a family environment it's..*

It's a given.

So for three quarters of the year,
full time,
I was having to
work at being loved.
Work at being good..
When I say being good,
I don't necessarily mean behaving,
but sort of working at
favour from..

Sue: from staff, or...

From staff, from other pupils..

Sue: Being accepted I suppose as well.

Yes.
Yes..
I suppose it changed as the weeks went on;
from quite an exciting thing,
to then......
thinking...
"this is just rubbish"

Tony also talks about his experience of education:

Tony: I started off at a school for the...
what used to be "special school" and
there it was
they just gave you work which was very undemanding
this was in the 50's.
Then I went to a secondary school
but the title for anyone with Cerebral Palsy or sight problems was

either "looney" or "spas".

These are terms which are not
which are occasionally used today, but not very often
that's where we have come on
But there is a still deep seated
view about people with disabilities,
and I'm using the wider term
there is not that depth of vision educationally
to viewing people on a par ….
Maybe it's partly due to us.
I readily admit that we're not very good at dealing with things
sometimes..
I'm not!

So really it's a learning curve,
and a doing curve.

Mike goes on to talk about his experience of education as a
graduate and post-graduate where he was often the only person
who was visually impaired:

Mike: It is interesting,
there is one really difficult experience that I remember;
I did struggle in that environment,
it wasn't as if I felt accepted by everybody,
I didn't feel not accepted,
but the more I think,
the more I remember,
there were lots of conversations about how I wanted to feel
included..
And how sometimes I didn't feel included at all.

I remember one particular person,
    and I was going into chapel,
    this was someone I knew very well,
and she was handing out the service books, or hymn books,
and she said,
"Here's yours".

I can't remember exactly what happened,
But I probably said something like,
"I don't need one".

I asked her afterwards about it and she said,
"well I don't think of you as any different than anyone else";
so that felt like a double issue,
because she had accepted me as part of the community,
and treated me exactly the same,
so it felt like the acceptance was not based on who I was,
but who perhaps..
she wanted me to be.

That's just a small example ...

Sue: But it's quite a big thing though?

Patrick emails me after hearing myself and Tony presenting some
of our stories at a counselling research conference:

Hi Sue and Tony,
Thank you for sharing so much at the conference last week. As I said
to you at the time your words completely took my breath away.

One of the challenges of blindness is you can never escape it. It
surrounds you all the time. You can never close your eyes and hope

that it goes away. I seem to spend all of my time missing the clues to life. People think I'm rude or don't listen because I often miss the meaning of what is being said.

What has helped over the years – especially as a child was being part of a blind culture. All my friends at school were the same and having no sight at all set us apart and gained us respect. We were the elite with no trying to get by as sighted. In retrospect, being at school and then college with blind people was the happiest time in my life. It was much harder when I had to start living and interacting with the sighted. Suddenly I felt less confident and sure of myself and who I was. I tend even now to gravitate toward my blind friends.

It's quite strange because seeing you both talking about your experiences, and Sue you asking me whether there was anything I wanted to say about my own experiences that would help sighted people to respect my difference I almost said, "no. This is my world and they are not welcome". But I realised that was a bit selfish, especially for people who are losing sight and trying to make sense of it. Sometimes their pain however is more than I can bear, it feels like they are saying what I have is useless.

I do think though that it is very difficult for anyone with sight to fully understand the blind world, because the very fact of having sight makes it impossible to enter. If you "look" all the time from the sighted world to the blind world then you are blind to what it is like. I suppose it is like me trying to sit down with a newspaper. I cannot ever hope to understand the contents by just feeling the texture and size of the paper and counting the pages! I think that there is something about difference in people that we have to respect. I'm not sure we can ever fully understand someone else's situation, but we can respect that they have a different take on life. Schooling seems the key. To be brought up with difference or with familiarity?

Employment rate amongst the population of working age people who are registered blind or partially sighted is estimated as 33% (Douglas et al. 2009) this is less than half the number of adults without a disability who are employed, and significantly less than groups of people with any other disability.

Several people contact me to talk about their experiences with employment. Tony talks about how the ongoing search for employment has affected his life:

Tony: I've always been a busy person in the past.
I've tried to be anyway!

Sue: It's that kind of purpose is really important,
Well it is to me,

because I've got what you call probably a
work ethic.

When I did work...
    I still want to work...as I've told you,
but after the workshop closed in Liberty Lane,
    I went there before I was diagnosed with serious eye problems,
but they had a mixture of people there,
people who were disabled, who were on the register.
I've been on the register for years and years and years,
    but my sight was better then.

Since I had that job,
which was in the early eighties,
    or the middle eighties,
(I can't quite remember the date,
    it's been closed now for quite a few years..)

A lot of people were disappointed in it,
    it was rather like a...
except for the people who worked there in managerial capacities,
    it was not particularly people friendly.
It was like a sweat shop.

They treated me alright,
the workers treated me alright,
and the office staff treated me alright,
but the managerial...not so much.

They couldn't make it commercially pay,
but they should have tried to adapt it,
    shouldn't they?
It was rather old fashioned in many ways.

Sue: but you enjoyed working there?

Well...
I enjoyed meeting the people,
the actual job was crap
    (excuse the French).

I was doing a job which as I've told you before
    was below my mental capacity,
I didn't mind doing it,
but it didn't stretch me at all.
That's why I used to have a chat to people
chat away to people, in the process of my job.
I used to ....
One of my jobs was cleaning the loos out,
    which I didn't mind,
but you can't clean them out every 10 minutes Can you?
It was very poorly structured,

in that what they brought out of people.
The people who did the skilled jobs were ..
   those of us who weren't doing skilled jobs,
   and I was really a labourer
..you know ..
nothing wrong with that ..
but they never asked you
whether you wanted to do anything else.

 ..I think they thought the writing was on the wall.

Sue: So it wasn't about empowering people?

Oh no, no ..it was very old fashioned.
Except though they had a union ..
but they never went on strike;
whereas I would have..
I did suggest,
"why don't you complain to management about the working conditions, and the fact that it might be closing",
and they said:
"Can't….
We'll Go back to our regional office and get their advice…"
They're quite entitled actually to decide themselves.

There was no empowerment as you say…
It was a job
and frankly you felt as if you were ..
had to feel as if you were jolly glad you were in an organisation like that!

Sue: What happened when it closed?
Well I was just out of work..
And then I got very depressed,
and then I had a breakdown.

Yes it's a common theme I'm afraid,
Trying to find employment or voluntary work.
And the thing is Sue..
when I went to the job centre they said,
"Oh you'll be alright…
now don't worry about work,
you know you're not capable of doing very much,
say that again?
"well…I'm capable of doing more than you think that I might be".
They didn't want the bother really.
Placing people.
Because most disability re-settlement officers,
well they used to be called that then,
are not really interested
in getting people with disabilities back into work,
if they can get one in…

Oh! (claps hands). Good for them!

It pays "Lip service".
They're not interested..
I mean they don't look for the best job suitable,
I mean they sent me to Remploy on one occasion,
this is regarding work,
and it was for a totally inappropriate work..

They told me to be there at 7 o'clock in the morning,
which was not easy!
(The other place I had to be there at 7.30 in the morning)

When I got there the bloke …
a sort of semi-supervisor sort of bloke,
he wasn't a manager,
with one of these brown coats,
said,
"what are you doing here?"
I said, "I've come here to work.
I like to be early".
He said "I told them not to send you 'til 9.00!"
He was very rude, and offensive).
I said,
"You behave like a fascist don't you?"
And I walked out.
I wasn't going to stand that.

He was Curt. Curt.
Rude, and curt.
I went back to tell them at the office that he had a very curt
demeanour,
and I told them that I thought that it was because they could get
away with that sort of thing..

Sue: It's being talked down to..

Exactly,
Or talked to; as if you're a piece of dirt
almost.
I mean, I took the trouble ..
and she said "don't worry Tony,
I know what they're like down there".

Well if she knew what they were like,
she shouldn't have sent me in the first place!

I guessed that it was part of her remit to send them anywhere.
(Laughter)
Years ago…years ago there was more opportunity,
in the 60's or 50's, for disabled people.
Because there were lift attendants and people like that,

they don't have those today do they?
There were jobs
they took it more seriously.
When I went to certain jobs they didn't take it seriously at all.

Sue: What's that like? I'm wondering what that has been like facing that attitude over and over again?

Not very good.
That's why I had a breakdown,
because, I was at home constantly thinking about that;
you know, being cowered down and rejected.
And although I've got a certain amount of strength,
In fact,
people tell me I've got a lot of
inner reserve which ..
They wonder how I haven't gone completely bonkers ..
I don't tell them I have been completely bonkers (laughter)
I haven't found it difficult, ever,
to get on with other members of staff.
It is the management ...the people who I find the most offensive are generally the management side,
who make decisions without consulting you.

Sue: You told me once about when you were working as a volunteer for Oxfam, how when the management changed attitudes changed?

I had to sit down, waiting for someone to supervise me.
Well **I wasn't** going to stand for that;
I'd done the job for 4 years, that's where I met (name deleted).
And she treated me like ..
If I fell down then I fell down and she helped me up,
and we got on.
That's where she was very good.
But, there's too much of this "politically correct"
"You can't do that, you can't do this".
Do you agree with me?

Sue: Yes. Absolutely. Because it's that kind of political correctness ..

Stultifying....
It comes under the label "health and safety";
do they think that everyone who falls down might sue them?
I never had any intention of suing them.

Maria emailed me in response to listening to Tony's story and tells of her own experiences of employment and learning:

Dear Sue,

Thank you for asking me to read some of the stories in your latest project.

As you know I have been visually impaired all my life, and also have mild cerebral palsy which has affected my speech and my ability to get about.

When I listened to your conversation with Tony, it brought tears to my eyes. His experiences so resonated with the battle I have had all my life, and how hard it has been to keep battling sometimes. I have often over the years debated whether life is really worth living, but have always managed somehow to keep going.

Feeling accepted for who I am though has always been a major issue.

I have never had a "proper" job. I have done so many training courses, that I am probably the most educated woman in the UK, and could paper my lounge with the certificates. But, despite this, and my applying for literally hundreds of posts (both voluntary and paid) I have never been considered suitable for any real job. People always assume that because of my disabilities I am unable to do anything but the most mundane of tasks.

When I say this I feel very sad, disappointed, and sometimes just bloody angry.

I have had some counselling in the past, but this just made me feel worse, because the counsellor told me that I should stop playing the "victim" and take responsibility for how I felt. This felt so unfair – it was like she was blaming me for other people's prejudices, and that I just had to accept my sad fate. It is a miracle I didn't physically assault her! I hasten to add that I never went back!

I am so glad that Tony was brave enough to say all these things, I think that unless we start talking about our experiences, however hard that is, then nothing will ever change.

You asked me how I thought my visual impairment affects my identity, and I am not sure how to answer this, except to say that the not seeing (although frustrating) does not affect me, but that other people's assumptions about me based on the fact that I am partially sighted and have a speech impediment make me feel worthless and useless and patronised. I have battled all my life with feeling accepted for who I am.

My friends and family however have been a tower of strength over the years, and their love has helped me to think that at least with them I am worth something, even if I do feel more than a bit of a burden at times.

Caroline has worked for the last 13 years in local government (since leaving university with a first class honours degree in business study) we met to talk about her experiences.

Caroline: Being at university was ok.
I finally felt as if I could get on with my life.
There was a certain amount of the normal hassle,
like tutors not remembering to give me
handouts in electronic format.

They would see me sitting in the class and then go into a major panic (even though I had been sitting in the same class all year). "Oh dear, I'll just run along to the office and see if they can do something with this stuff for you".
Pitiful really, but I got by.

There were all the usual crass comments like
"I'm really sorry" "it must be so difficult" "what a shame"
but most of my mates knew I could down the beers like the best of them!

Working for a local authority has had its ups and downs,
They have provided accessible software for my computer, and nearly always remember to give me things in the right format,
but it is assumed ..
It is assumed that I will never be suitable for promotion,
I do the mundane clerical tasks that no-one else wants to do.

I get so frustrated sometimes
because I am just sidelined by people.
My opinion does not matter.
Several years ago I took out a grievance against my manager because she never included me in team meetings or decisions and although I won the grievance, and moved teams, the kind of covert discrimination still goes on.
I have decided now not to fight it.
If I fought for my rights all the time I would burn out!

I do other things in my spare time
currently I am doing a masters with the OU.
I can see why blind people enjoy being academics!

Working as an academic is indeed easier because very often mobility is not an issue, and if I am writing academic papers those reading them will not know about my visual impairment unless I tell them. Presenting papers at conferences is very challenging and often leaves me physically shaking. Using accessible technology in front of an audience is fraught with danger and gives an added anxiety. Being seen to struggle publicly is not something many of us would choose, but something that is part and parcel of the experience of being visually impaired. John Hull writes of his own experiences as an academic who regularly gave lectures and talks:

> "I tried dictating to myself by making a recording of the whole speech, or a summary and using an earplug. For a while I actually tried to listen and speak at the same time, but after one or two disastrous experiences I gave this up. I tried using Braille headings. This not only involved laborious preparation, but my Braille was just not good enough. I could not scan quickly enough to get myself out of the difficulty which arose when I forgot what to say next." (Hull 1990:201)

Hull found that if he put aside assumptions (based I feel on sighted concepts that we need some kind of visual clue to enable us to speak publicly) and just "spoke" as if in normal conversation then he was very successful.

> "Somehow or other, and without effort, I have developed a way of scanning ahead in my mind, to work out what I am going to say." (Hull 1990:201)

Employment statistics are often misleading, but in this case perhaps reflect societal attitudes that people with a visual impairment could not possibly succeed in doing work that involves visual processes. What it fails to recognise is that people who are visually impaired are often very skilled and adept at developing new and creative ways of achieving the same outcomes, as in the case of public speaking. John Hull is an inspirational speaker!

The etiquette of the sighted (Part Four)

It is sometimes taken as "truth" that the visual is the dominant construct through which we accumulate knowledge and present this knowledge to others, both within academia and in wider communities. Thinking of this for a moment from a post-structuralist position, then perhaps this "visual" is not "the truth" but one of many different possibilities, and to enable "blind" researchers to be able to "observe" and "read" and be taken seriously then the discourses surrounding visual "truth" would need to be deconstructed.

An interesting academic discourse took place between two philosophers Magee and Milligan (1995), the latter being blind, on whether as Magee thought, lack of sight limited people in the development of a phenomenology because, he felt, the primary sense by which one gathers information was lost. Milligan was a member of the American National Federation of the Blind, and considered that the world could be communicated and understood through other senses. The interchange was fascinating, but unfortunately was terminated on the death of Milligan however, it highlighted the prevalence of the assumption especially within academia that the world can only be assimilated through the visual, so those of us who are visually impaired are therefore "less able".

Reading and text are seen as the primary ways in which we accumulate knowledge. What is reading though? Do you agree with Wilemans (1980) definition "seeing with the eyes and understanding that which is seen" (Wileman 1980:12; cited by Kinash 2005:14) or Kinash's own definition, "deciphering symbols to attain meaning" (Kinash 2005:14)? Where I wonder does that leave the high percentage of visually impaired people who do not read Braille? After all, 90% become blind over the age of 60 (RNIB 2008) and Braille requires dexterity of touch that many have by then lost. What about those who are reliant on audio, or who, like me, often access text via a text-reader. Are we readers? Sadly there is not sufficient room within this book to consider the complexities of this question, but I would be interested to know whether you are currently choosing to "read" the print version of this book, or "listen to" the audio, and the reasons for your choice.

I am able to read text, but I often find that it is being provided in too small print for me to comfortably read. The most amusing example was when I was presenting at a recent diversity conference about "the emotional responses to sight loss, and the need for accessible practices", where all the programme information was given to me in very small print. When I pointed this out the comment was made "I'm so sorry, I had you down as a presenter not a V.I.P. (Visually impaired person)". Words failed me on that occasion, but I do think that it highlights the expectation that people who "present research to others" or academics are not V.I.P's!

Following a presentation of some of these stories at a conference I meet with Emma who is in her thirties and has been visually impaired all her life:

Emma: I got through university by being bolshie!
"she's the blind girl with attitude"
I was always the one, who partied the hardest,
took the toughest subjects,
got the highest grades,
and joined the most way out societies (like bungee jumping).

I had learnt through school that to survive meant throwing off
"victim status"
otherwise you got nowhere.

I was recruited by one of the big insurance companies graduate
schemes.
They made no bones about the fact that I would have to
"keep up or get out".

It was so tough though –
constantly changing locations,
I'd just about get my head around the routes around one town and
then I'd be moved to another.
I had to give presentations from memory
(couldn't read my notes)
Manage a team twice my age
(who thought that not seeing meant they could get away with stuff)
I started drinking heavily to get myself through,
and it came to a head when at a really important deal I turned up
after I had drunk half a bottle of whisky and…

I broke down in front of everyone.

That was it.
Downward spiral until I left.
Now I'm on benefit.
That really sucks.
Receiving handouts,
Afraid that everything will change at the whim of the government.
I have now enrolled at college and am determined to start again
The bastards will not grind me down!

Will emails me from Aukland New Zealand:

Hi Sue
I've always worked, or tried to!. Since college where they expected
us all to be piano tuners! I decided to be a community worker, and
did my stint at university. After a long time of searching I finally
came across the family centre in Adelaide. Since then I have
worked in many therapeutic settings mainly with young people
involved with the DHS. I love my work and have never found my
sight an issue – except with the management who at times are
bloody minded and discriminatory.

Michael also emails me regarding work and benefits:

Hi Sue,
I suppose what I would like to add to those who suggest that people
on benefits are milking the system is:

Do you know what it's like to not have a job?
Never to be considered worthy of paid employment?
To always be on benefits,
always afraid of government cutbacks
Apologising for going on holiday.
Always offered training and never opportunities to use the training!

CHAPTER FIVE

AM I GOING MAD?

Chapter Five explores the experience of living with visual hallucinations and societal attitudes which link losing sight with deteriorating mental health. Although visual hallucinations are not widely known about, contributors felt that they had a huge impact on their life and how they perceived their identity, and there is still little written about this common phenomenon. The chapter also explores current literature relating to visual hallucinations and "Charles Bonnet Syndrome".

Sarah talks about the visual hallucinations she sees:

Sarah[1] The angels.
The angels appear again
"do not be troubled" they say.
All I can see sometimes is their sad eyes.

I spent about six months wanting to die
but the angels kept coming,
crying in my eyes.

I've had my life,
now I want to die.

Last year when he (husband) died
My first thought was "freedom".
Then the angels came.
Guilt came on me
weighed me down.

My first thought when I knew he was gone was "freedom",
so much of the world to see,
even going out to the bingo without his voice
shouting in my face.

Then the angels came
"gambling is the devils work" he would have said.

Him dying seemed to open the gate for me – I stood on the threshold

---

[1] Excerpts from this story were first published in (Dale 2008c)

Then the angels danced in my eyes.
He took my sight and sent me the angels to spy.

Now I have discovered that my angels are not madness
they are shadows;
many people have them
the brain tries to make up for not seeing.
No-one told me,
I thought I was going mad
But angels they are, and they haunt me.

Chris emails me after listening to Sarah's story at a workshop. Like Sarah she knew nothing about Charles Bonnet syndrome and was too frightened to talk to anyone about what she was experiencing:

Hi Sue,
When you get to a certain age you start to worry about dementia. It's probably our worst fear; losing your mind and other people taking over your life.

My mother had Alzheimer's so after my sixtieth birthday I started to watch myself, to keep a record of when I forgot things or forgot where I had put them. I lost a lot of my sight quite suddenly when I was sixty five. I had what was supposed to have been fairly routine eye surgery that turned into a nightmare. Losing sight was traumatic. I went from someone who was a "helper" and community driver to one of those who was "helped". The frustration of doing even simple tasks was extreme. I remember one day being picked up by a friend to go shopping and not being able to find the list that I had so carefully made. I tore the kitchen apart looking for it, and when my friend arrived there was chaos – things everywhere and me just weeping uncontrollably. She was very kind, but didn't, couldn't comprehend why I was so upset. "You only had to wait until I came, the list is here in the hall, where you left it".

When I was lying in bed, first thing in the morning, I would often open my eyes and see my mother calmly sitting in the rocking chair by the dressing table – she had been dead for over twelve years by this time. Other times a fleeting image of a cat stalked me. Sometimes worms erupted from the sink or even my dinner. I was scared. Was this what it was like to go mad?

I felt I couldn't trust anything or anyone. I remember my GP asking how I was coping at home. "Fine" I said "absolutely fine". I was afraid of two things; that he would say I needed to go into a home, and that he would tell me that dementia was not the end of the world. I knew that it was. If I could just keep these images at bay then I would be ok.

Then some years later I went to a workshop at the local "blind club" (yeuch what a terrible name) and one lady was calmly talking about visual hallucinations and how she saw shadows of people when they were not there. She said she had looked it up on the macular society's web site and that these were a normal side effect of sudden sight loss. I told her about my mother. "You've got this Charles Bonnet thing too" she said. At my next hospital appointment I asked the doctor about it, and he confirmed that many people were affected by visual disturbances following sight loss. The feeling sitting there was elation, I was not going mad, then anger. Why was I not warned it might happen?

Beth sends me a poem about the images that she sees:

Colours for a Blind Woman
Blue
Red
Black
Swirling dervishes
Blue
Red
Black
Moving in your face as I look at you
Blue
Red
Black
Haunting me, Taunting me
Blue
Red
Black
Walking down the street
Blue
Red
Black
No Escape
Blue
Red
Black
Close my eyes
Orange
Orange
Orange

So often we consider that "truth" is only something that we can see and we are reliant on visual images to help us determine reality from fiction. What happens to our sense of self and reality therefore when we start seeing things that are not there? Phil emails me pondering on this very question:

Hi Sue,

There is something about seeing equating to truth. If I see something with my own eyes then I know it exists. What does this mean I wonder if I see something that is not there? I often see a dog lying by the fire. He gives me great comfort, but if I reach out to touch him he moves out of my sight. He watches me peacefully and I am calmed by his acceptance and presence. I know that he is not "real" in the sense of a physical animal that needs food and walking. I talk to him sometimes as I would to a pet. Does this mean I am losing my grip on sanity? I know that the hallucinations are normal for someone such as myself who has lost sight over a relatively short period of time, but when I start using those hallucinations to self-soothe is that stepping too far into a non-reality?

Somehow losing my sight has meant that I go more and more inwards towards this kind of internal world that is so different and alien from any of my sighted friends and family. The dog is sometimes more real to me than my friends who prattle on about "this and that" in their sighted world and who feel so far away because I cannot see their faces or their expressions.

Don't worry Sue, I'm not expecting you to give me any answers! It helps to share these thoughts with others who may be interested.

Beth follows up her poem with an email:

Hi Sue,

Unlike many people I did get told about Charles Bonnet Syndrome some years ago when I talked to my counsellor at the RNIB. This did dispel some of my fears. I have been seeing these images now for a long time, and although I am not frightened by them in the way that others describe, I do find them increasingly tedious and exhausting. Whatever I'm doing they are there wildly going round and round. I find it very hard to use my residual vision because of the flashing colours and lights.

Someone asked me at the eye clinic what was the worst bit about losing my sight and she was very surprised when I told her that it was the intrusive visual images! Somehow when someone is registered blind you don't expect them to complain about what they can see, more about what they can't.

It is also difficult to talk to friends and family about these images, they tend to think that I am going (or already) mad. There is just so much that my sighted friends do not understand, and sometimes it is too wearying to talk to them about it.

Pauline also emailed me after listening to Sarah's story with her own experiences of visual hallucinations:

Hello Susan,

I listened to Sarah's story and I had to write to firstly thank Sarah for telling her story so eloquently and for being brave enough to start talking about issues which are not talked about even within eye clinics.

Sarah talked about seeing angels and how these affected her life and how she thought she was going mad. **Why don't people warn you about Charles Bonnet Syndrome??**

I am 64 and was diagnosed with dry AMD in one eye and wet in the other. This meant injections of Lucentis for one eye, but nothing for the other. I had four monthly appointments at my local eye clinic, the injections made little difference and my sight continued to deteriorate. After my second injection I woke one morning and discovered to my horror what looked like blood dripping through the ceiling. I shot out of bed shaking. When I looked at the ceiling again it had gone. I put it down to being half asleep, but it was the beginning of a really bizarre time. I started to see images everywhere – faces coming through the walls, snakes erupting from the carpet, psychedelic patterns. I was frightened. I rang the eye clinic who advised me they couldn't bring my appointment forward and suggested I go to my GP. He was useless, had never heard of anything like it. He asked me whether I was experiencing acute anxiety or depression "Of course I'm anxious" I said "so would you be with snakes coming out of the floor!". He offered me a course of anti-depressants, but this didn't seem like the right answer. He referred me to see a psychiatrist. The psychiatrist thought that perhaps the shock of sight loss had caused psychosis and put me on a course of anti-psychotic medication. This did help me feel a bit calmer, but did nothing to halt the faces and coloured patterns which swirled through my life. He did say he wondered if this might be something to do with my vision problem and advised I speak to my ophthalmologist. Again the eye clinic could not offer an appointment (they had recently sent a letter putting back my quarterly appointment by a month. The receptionist suggested if I was really concerned that I go to A & E. I felt so desperate that I did. I waited several hours and finally was seen by this charming young doctor who said "I don't think it's anything to worry about, it is probably just Charles Bonnet Syndrome". That was how I found out. It was such a relief just to know what was causing the problem. I didn't have schizophrenia or Alzheimer's! It was just a reaction to sight loss. The very worse thing about it all was the not knowing.

The images have faded over time, they still pop up occasionally, but on the whole they don't worry me so much.
I really think that people should be warned about this though. I don't want others to go through what I did!

Charles Bonnet Syndrome was named after a Swiss philosopher when he described this condition in 1760. Despite the passage of time however there is still little known about the causes of these hallucinations (Schadlu, Schadlu, and Shepherd 2009) and only limited treatment possibilities (Eperjesis and Akbarali 2009; Batra, Bartels, and Wormstall 2009). Little information is still given to patients who are likely to experience the symptoms and many general practitioners and high street optometrist who have never heard of it. It was thought to be rare, but a review by Rovener (2006) suggested that Charles Bonnet Syndrome "will affect an increasingly large number of older persons as the population ages and the occurrence of vision and cerebral disorders increases" (Rovener 2006:275). Organisations such as the RNIB and the Macular Society are working to ensure both eye care professionals and individuals affected by sight loss are aware of the syndrome and how it affects people[2]. What seems apparent when talking to the contributors of this book is that knowing about the syndrome has taken away a lot of the fears and anxieties and that the hallucinations have had less affect on their lives. Sarah sends me a poem:

> Angels take flight
> their judgement dispelled
> how knowledge disperses their power.
> They can come now
> I do not despair
> they are wisps of nothing
> beneath my blind gaze
> they fade
> not important
> not needed
> the end.

---

[2] for more information about Charles Bonnet Syndrome see www.macularsociety.org or www.rnib.org

PART 2

LIVING LIFE AS SOMEONE
WHO IS BLIND OR PARTIALLY SIGHTED

Chapter Six

Societal Attitudes towards Blindness

In Chapter One there was a discussion about public perceptions of blindness and how this differs from an individual's experience of living with a visual impairment. This chapter expands on this theme, and considers how societal attitudes affect the self and identity. It also explores "visual truth" compared with socially constructed identity and the first part of the commentary entitled: "re-authoring blindness"

Journal 4 November 2008

Walking this morning I think about Mike's words, and his desire to "walk in the sky". Because of the low winter sun, there is a luminous quality in the heavens above me. I can see clouds lined with pink and silver, and a buzzard as he glides effortlessly across the sky.

I look down. It is like looking from heaven to hell, the grass, mud, stones, branches all tangle together in swathes of dark shadows, which I cross with trepidation.

*I've been thinking a lot too about **passivity**. As visually impaired people, do we always have to be passive recipients of life? **Of course not. Never, but,** when you cannot see the other person, or their face, the world about you has to reach out and touch you, or you have to stumble into it before you can react. It is very difficult to reach out and touch something you don't know exists. How do you know when to speak, to wave, to cross the room to avoid the party bore?*

***Passivity**, rather like **gratitude** is something that is expected of people who are blind or partially sighted. It is also a pragmatic response I adopt which enables life to proceed without too much hassle and anguish.*

Sometimes though, I have the feeling of life rushing past me, and I am only able to catch a little of it as I hold my hands out blindly. But doing this is sometimes hazardous, instead of my hands touching against angels' wings they sometimes get caught against thorns!

Often my conversations with people are about their feelings of being patronised and how that makes them feel "less than normal" (Andy). My conversations with Tony have often been about social injustice and how societal attitudes affected his, and other people's lives. Here we join one of our many conversations about this subject, talking specifically about the attitudes of the organisations that are set up to support people who are visually impaired:

Tony: People speak to you as if you are a non-entity

Sue: It's about being patronised?

Tony: Patronised is the right word.
I don't know whether during your work
lots of people feel patronised?

Sue: Yes.

Patronised is one of the big feelings I have sometimes.

They are "very nice',
 but I don't want people to be, "very nice",
I want them to be, "very effective".
I want them to be
just natural.
Not "Alright? How are you today" (in nice voices).
"Everything alright... Good..".

Sue: that doesn't leave you space.....

It's **throttling.**

Starving.

That's all I want really,
I don't want a lot of extra....

Normal.

I want to be treated like a normal person.
Having some control, by the way;
as we've discussed before,
and not feeling as if ..
as an example,
this week for instance..
the bloke from the agency
who provide support for me,
he was the project director..

He phoned me up and said,
"do you mind somebody coming at 12.30?"
I said, "I do, yes...
really,
Because I stipulated that I like to see my people,
my person in the morning..
Because I don't want to be in all day".

Maybe some days I want to be in,
but just to say it out of the blue..

Then about ten minutes later he phoned me up again
and said,
"Rachel will be coming on Tuesday".
And I said "Oh yes?"
(I had never heard of Rachel)
and then,
"does this mean that Sam's not coming again?"
(Sam is my regular worker)
he said "I've got a different plan for Sam".

When Sam came with Rachel ..
they both came together,
I said,
"Is that right,
you're leaving me?
what happened?..
you didn't say a word to me".

It's very wrong,
he didn't give her the chance to tell me herself.
(She was angry with him),
and said,
"I would have been able to explain to you the reason",
he didn't explain,
just said that he had plans for her;
as if she were a performing donkey...

Sue: It's treating people like commodities ..

Yes. Commodities..
when she came she said,
"I'm very annoyed with him".
I said, "so was I".
She knew I was annoyed,
not with her.
I said,
"This is not you,
you probably didn't know about it".

She said,
"I wanted to be able to tell you myself".

Which she proceeded to do.
Which he didn't give her the opportunity to do.

Sue: but it doesn't give you any voice at all in this, does it?

I have got absolutely no voice
with these organisations they ..
I asked him,
"Have you taken up my suggestion
about getting a client council?"
"No-one is interested" he said...

No they won't be unless you ask!

I'm interested because I want to help run this company;
in a sort of ideas way.
It calls itself a charity but ..
they charge enough!...
(laughter)
I thought to myself after speaking to him;
"what a ...rather bizarre way of conducting things!"

Mo also speaks of her experiences of interacting with agencies set up to support people who are visually impaired:

Mo: I had a volunteer
which I suppose I had to be grateful for,
she was very nice,
but always talked to me like I was 5!

"Do you want to go to the park today dear?"

For God's sake!

The (organisation name deleted) was much better,
some people there actually talked to me as if I was a human being,
but there was still something of that attitude.

Them and Us.

"we are ok" (sighted)
"you need caring for" (blind)
It just makes me feel so, so useless and hopeless.

As stated earlier there are many societal assumptions about what being registered as blind mean, and these assumptions become part of what is offered to people in the way of support, and this support does not always tie up with what is actually needed. Dennis talks here about his experiences of walking with a group set up to assist people who are visually impaired:

Dennis: Visually impaired people were paired up with sighted people so..
whoever got the blind guy they knew where they were at,
because the blind guy would hold their arm
and they would need a dialogue as to what was coming up
climbing over stiles, going through a field, in the woods, or whatever.

But of course someone that gets me
doesn't know where they are ..
they haven't got a clue.

"How can I help you?.."
"You can't
just tell me if there's an unusual hazard, or if there is something coming up".

But it wasn't even that,
it was the fact of how the leader of the group
sort of assumed responsibility for all of us,
which is ...is laudable!
I mean he feels responsible,
but **we are adults**.

Sue: Yes but he's kind of ...
it's being turned into child like ..

Well it is,
because, I had my designated helper
and we actually got separated.
And I'm not going to look out for him,
and think, "am I following him everywhere?"
I was with a couple of other folk who were "spare" sighted people
and they were friends, and suddenly I found myself ..

We were in a town,
and the group leader was marching back towards me and he said to me,

"Dennis we've been looking for you"

and I said "well here I am. What's the problem?"

"Alan has lost you".

"No. No" I said
"Alan hasn't lost me, we got separated".

"But you've got to stay with him"

"Well its not my fault if he wanders off!"
"Well you've just got to ..
you know ...

not get lost"
basically.

Alan came back,
and I started chatting with him and he said to me,
"I was worried we were going to have to ring your wife and say
we've lost you".
And I said,
"can you hear yourself?
I have travelled all over the world by myself. We are in a town in
England
I've got …
I know how phones work,
if I got lost,
do you not think I could sort myself out?"

"Well I wasn't sure …"
he bumbled and mumbled a bit ..
and I just thought,

"I don't know whether I want to be here?
I don't know if I can handle this?"

And this was the same group
that when we took a wrong turn
they knocked on the door, and the guy was a bit unfriendly;
    maybe tourists knocked on the door a lot
but one of our group;
the guy wouldn't straight away say, "you've got to go this way or
that way"
because they told him where they wanted to go
but one of the guys, who was **my friend** said,
    I didn't hear him say it, but he told me afterwards said to him,
"we've got some blind people with us
and **they are starting to get upset"**.

Sue: Sigh!

And I just..

Sue: But it's the whole attitude …

Oh yes, oh yes.

Sue: "got to be taken care of",
looked after.

I challenged him.
I challenged him about this
but I did it in a very kind of tactful way.
I didn't say, "that's wrong"
I actually said to him..

I didn't say anything at the time..
but when we were on the way home
we were in a car, a day or so later,
We were talking about the whole weekend
and I said,
"do you ever think about the way you handle visual impaired people?
I know you do it a lot.
Do you ever think you get it wrong?"
He said, "no".
I thought, "fine
a lost cause".

Sue: I was remembering something.....
One of the things that really gets to me
is when people say something about
"we've got to do this for the blind".

The blind

Sue: Perhaps they might add "the blind people"
I remember an incident where someone was reading through
something that I had written and she said: "what's all this about
people who consider themselves blind or partially sighted?
What does that mean?
They're either blind or they're not!"

Laughter

Sue: And I said ..
"No it's not quite like that".
I could feel myself getting angry.
I was beginning to get a bit angry about this..
"Actually", I said
*"I consider myself a **person**.*
Being blind or partially sighted,
*   which is where I put myself,*
*is **only part of who I am**, it is not all of me!"*

Yes.
It's that assumption again.

Sue: But she wouldn't have it.
You're a different race. If you're blind you're blind.

Yes. That's what we need to challenge.

Sue: That's the challenge isn't it?

Yes. **Big time**.
Oh Big time.

I don't go walking with them anymore.

Which is sad.
But I can't take the patronisation.
I just can't.

I can't handle it.

I'm convinced that they think that it is me that has got the problem.
I'm convinced of it.

I really am.
That's what really frustrates me
when people say,
"it's because of your sight problem".

"You're angry because of your sight problem"
you know, "you're frustrated because of your sight problem"
and It's not quite as straight forward as that.

Sue: It's about attitudes?...

It's about the way one is being treated.
That's right.

Re-authoring blindness (Part One)

Traditional psychological theories (Maslow 1968, 1973; Rogers 1961, 1978; Mower 1962) would have us believe that "who we are" is something found within. If we look hard enough, and peel off enough layers, we can grow, actualize, and discover our "real self" (Rowan 1983). Within the latter half of the 20th century and the beginning of the 21st century, people have taken time out of community to "find themselves", and the counselling and therapeutic industries have encouraged us to shut out the demands of the outside world, and look within our own life for meaning and identity. I have as a counsellor both encouraged others, and personally explored my inner world of thoughts, feelings, and behaviours, with very rich results.

However, if we for a moment examine identity from a postmodern perspective, and start to look at it as something that is socially constructed (Freedman and Combs 1996), then we can see that a sense of self is not just an internal reality, but actually created through relationship within the society we live and by the stories we tell to ourselves and others to make sense of our lives. My questions however are, that if the society that we have relationship with considers that the main way of communicating our identity is visual, and that sighted is normal, and blind is definitely not normal, then what does that mean for those of us who are visually impaired, and how we negotiate our identity? And, if we as people who are blind or partially sighted (which puts us very much in the minority) constantly come up against what I have described in previous chapters as "the etiquette of the sighted", how does this affect how we feel about ourselves. As Hull so eloquently writes:

> "What affects me is the cumulative experience of the inescapable presence of blindness. Perhaps it is also the lack of control, and this may well be why I find it so exhausting… The social demands of public life and the personal demands of family life seem to create so many situations in which I become not only aware but painfully aware of blindness". (Hull 1990:92).

Even if we do not "lose" sight and we are not affected by the overwhelming emotional turmoil that "loss" (especially that of a sense) entails. We will inevitably come up against the societal norm which relies on visually constructed truth. Our transport, employment, communication and even academic systems consider that "sight" is a vital element of that system and it is unimaginable for many to consider negotiating any of them without sight. For example within the UK most adults drive, and it is both a symbol of status, and convenient for accessing work, leisure and shopping facilities. Those who do not drive are relegated often to second rate public transport systems that do not enable people to travel beyond the borders of cities and large urban areas. Even public transport systems such as trains and busses are not necessarily easy to use with low vision.

The following conversation with Dennis highlights some of the issues regarding transport, but also importantly demonstrate how societal attitudes regarding what it means to be blind affects him:

Dennis: It's about …
choices…
do I use the white cane or don't I use the white cane?
For example:
I've got to get a train….

I'm in Sheffield,
the journey there was planned well,
but I've got to get back to Sheffield station.

And obviously because I came out of Euston which I know really well,
that didn't hold any fears for me,
but I know I've got to get back to Sheffield station and get the train home,
and I noticed when I came in to Sheffield
that it is quite a complicated station.
So, I've got two choices:

Either:
Take the white cane out and go straight to the information desk
and say, "can you find someone to help me?"
Or:

Do I leave the white cane in my bag,
and get my monocular out, and try to read the indicator board?

And as I even think about that;
I feel very differently
between those two particular ways of dealing with this.

The one with the white cane and asking for help..
"fraud" starts to come in;
because it's going to be worrying about
their assumptions that I am blind,
and yet, I am not.

And one can't suddenly
deliver my story to this individual,
who's probably busy anyway,
but they do tend to make assumptions,
or that's my fear.

Immediately they're going to be;
"I'll carry your bag".
So even if I say, "I prefer to carry it"
"No. I'll carry it"
Oh God....

"Do you need to hold my arm?"
"No thank you".

But then when I say no thank you,
I then feel
compelled to explain.

I can't just say "no thank you".
Because, if I do,
I will then be in this world of absolute anxiety,
that as I'm walking up the steps,
down the other side,
they're going to be thinking:

"I thought he was blind?
He's negotiated those stairs fine".

So that's where the fraud bit comes in.
And that's just the tip of the iceberg with that situation,
because I think that situation will often depend on;
"whoever" is giving me that assistance.

That's about them as a person, or personality,
I've had such varying experiences,
from somebody who's wonderful;
    and I'd love for them to be there every time,
to somebody who makes me feel like a package;
    that just had to be dealt with..

Sue: dispatched?

Got out of the way.
That was one choice. With the other one;

I guess with the other one I could still be holding the white cane..
but I'd need about three arms
because I'm holding my bag,
I'm getting my monocular out,
    which needs to be operated with two hands
in order to try and look at the indicator board.

But I know, even before I am going to take that avenue of dealing
with it;
that I'm going to get anxious,
because everything now is much slower,
so I have to allow a lot more time,
and of course the likelihood is that
the indicator board will say:

"London Euston",
and the time,
but the platform is not up yet.
So….I've then got to stand there,
and keep looking with my monocular,
waiting for the platform …

And because of the complexities of
Sheffield station;
because I can't read all the varying signs.
How do I find the platform?
Do I get there by getting it wrong,
by trial and error?
And I have done that before!
And if there's loads of time..
I suppose the thing is, if I am going to go down that avenue,
I have to allow a lot more time to get to the station.

Sue: There's still anxiety….

With the information desk route;
it's also important to emphasise…

About …

Relinquishing control.

What does it feel like to relinquish control?
and I can tell you,
it feels, bloody horrible.
you just feel;

"I'm useless".

It makes one feel useless
just to give that control over.
You're giving it over to somebody that could actually
show a fair amount of apathy.
They could be....

Sue: Brilliant?

or "Get out of the way because I'm busy"
   And yet really...
   Why can't they..?
I **should** be able to deal with either.
When I actually undertook that journey
I chose the "white cane" method
and it was ok,
I was taken to a waiting room,
and told:
"your train's going to be about 20 minutes.
I'll come back".

Sue: and there's fear there?

What if they forget?
And of course the announcements keep coming up
And I think,
If they **don't come back**
and the train's announced
I'm just going to...

Talk to anyone around me and say,
"look I can't see,
can you tell me where that train is?"

The point here is...

you're still living with the anxiety,
it's there all the time.

It is there all the time.

*Sue: It's handing over of responsibility to someone else,
you don't know who they're going to be,
you don't know whether you can trust them.*

Yes that's right.
I just feel very sensitive towards their attitude towards me,
   and yet **why** do I do that?

Why should I do that?

Would it be easier for me if I were a bit more "thick skinned",
and it didn't matter to me?

Should it matter to me?

And for some reason it does.

I suppose it is about
wanting to feel **good** about myself,

and I feel better about myself if they're a friendly soul,
and ask questions,
and I feel worse about myself
if they're off-hand;
   and make loads of assumptions.
And yet there is nothing I can do about that until the person in question
turns up.
I suppose
what it suggests to me that should rail staff have awareness training
for visually impaired people.

Sue: It's that giving up responsibility…
It's giving over of something that's….

Precious to me.

Even if I go to a station I know really well,
and I don't need help to find the platform,
and I don't need help to find the train,
because I am very familiar with ..
or the platform numbers are very big.
I still look at the train;
   and I've pre-looked at my ticket,
   pre-memorised my seat number,
   and coach number.
And I look at this train and I think:
It is going to be **such hard work** to find my seat.
It is going to be so much simpler to just say to somebody;

"Can you help me find my seat please?"

But again kicks in this business of having to explain.

Why do I do that?

Why do I say,
"I've got central vision blindness.
    It means that I can't see fine detail,
    I can see the train,
    but I can't read the platform numbers,
    and I can't read the carriage number,
    I can't read the number on the seat".

I find myself going through all of this;
time and time again,
and I feel "this is so wearying.
They must be tired of hearing it".
I have tried on a couple of occasions..
I've put my strong magnifier on
    which we are told we shouldn't walk around in,
but I sort of balance it on the end of my nose
on the train,
and I've gone along
and I've picked up the reservation tickets,
and looked at each one,
but very quickly a queue builds up behind you,
or someone will come up and want to get by
and you're peering at it ..
I just feel under such pressure,
that the next time I've got to do it,
I just think,
"don't put yourself through that".
Just give over the control for a little while
that's the best you're ever going to get.

Sue: so is it a relief when you do that?
Or is that worse?

No it's **not** a relief,
this is the problem,

it's not.

I suppose there is a sense of relief,
there is a sense of relief that I can just find what I want.
What is the quickest way to get what I want
and keep as much of my own self-esteem and control in place.
That's what I'm always looking for.
And yet there's always an element of;
everybody else can just look after themselves,
I **have** to seek help.

And I don't think that I'll ever be able to fully come to terms
with that aspect of travelling,
but,
you can't just let it bug you,
you just have to accept it

so I just try and..
laugh at it
I suppose.

Sarah emailed me following reading some of the stories from my doctoral project, including the excerpt from my conversation with Dennis shown above.

Dear Sue,
Thank you so much for including me in this project!

It feels so amazing to be on the receiving end of other people's stories instead of them giving feedback on mine.

Life has moved on so much from when we wrote the knitting stories, and I am so, so glad that they have been useful to others, and indeed I went to a local mothers' union to give a talk a few weeks ago, and someone said to me "I've just been on a course at the RNIB and listened to some stories which were absolutely amazing" what a small world! I didn't tell her it could have been my story she listened to!

When I read your conversation with Dennis I **felt so much.** So much of many different feelings. **Anger** – I am still so angry with hospitals for treating us in such an appalling way, and then **real empathy** for this "fraud" feeling. I have it all the time when I am out and about, and when I have to explain to people about my sight.

When Dennis spoke about the decisions of whether to use the white cane or not I could feel within myself exactly the same dilemma for which there is no answer, because either answer is wrong, and there is no escape. I then **laughed and laughed** until I thought I would never stop at his description of his peering at the seat reservations on the train through a magnifier, and the queue building up behind him. I think the laughter was the relief of knowing someone else had the same kind of problems and issues, sometimes this wretched eye condition makes me feel so very lonely. It also brought back memories of a journey I took at the end of the summer, I was doing really well, had got on the right train, found my seat, next to someone who I thought I recognised, and we talked throughout the journey (about an hour and a half) and as I was getting off he said: "It has been very interesting meeting you, but I think that you have mistaken me for someone else". I was so embarrassed, so ashamed. **Why did he not say something?** I wished that I could sink through the floor out of sight.

I am sure **it is right** for us to talk openly about our experiences, however hard that feels, because it is only by putting our voices together we can hope to change anything or anyone. Please thank Dennis Mike Adam and Tony for me for sharing these details of their lives!

Andy also responds to reading Dennis and Mike's story:

Hi Sue,
Reading through the stories I felt so much. Privileged to hear such amazing journeys! Angry with a world that just doesn't appreciate that sight is not always the truth of everything. Glad that there are other people out there who are visually impaired and live good rich lives. Amazed at how lucid and able you are all at articulating how you feel and think.

It took me back to thinking about my grandfather. He was a remarkable man, who died when I was about 9.

I remember though that I used to follow him around the garden as a small child, helping with the weeding, digging beside him with my small spade. He was a great story-teller, and told me tales about his life when he was my age. His favourite though was about his trips to the swimming pool, and the high dive platform.

My grandfather had polio when he was a small infant, and this had affected his legs badly. He walked always with a pronounced limp with the aid of callipers.

In the summer however he used to go with his friends to the outdoor lido, where there was a high dive platform. He used to take his callipers off and drag himself up the 8 flights of steps and then edge himself to the very end of the spring-board. By this time he had usually been noticed by the adults below. He could see people looking up at him and whispering, gesticulating for him to come down. He would stand, poised, for as long as he could on the end of the board, sensing the gasps from below him, before diving into the water.
He used to say,

> "imagine it. Me a cripple. Standing on that top board. Everyone thinking I would surely kill myself, and that they knew what was best for me. Then diving through the air – free as a bird. The only time I could ever prove the bastards wrong".

Why am I telling you this?

I suppose it is because as a child I never really understood what he meant, but now, through the experience of losing my sight, and telling my own story, and listening to other people's stories of being different, and coping not only with the challenges this difference brings, but other people's attitudes that try to contain me, keep me safe. I kind of understand because I feel free to be me when I write. Free as a bird, about the only time I do! Like my grandfather diving into the water below. And "me" is so much more than any disability.

Adam continues to explore how relationships with people who are sighted affect his sense of identity:

Adam: The other issues which feel very present for me at the moment
where I am today
is regarding control,
and how ...
I'll be absolutely honest I do not feel as if I have as much control,
as lots of other people that I know in my life,
and I don't have the same choices and control,
and I find that very difficult
and that has impacted on me and does impact on me in certain ways
and I'm really starting to learn that now.
I wouldn't necessarily describe myself as a "control freak"

Sue: I think we all like a degree of control in our life
lives and destiny!

But,
what I realise is that because
for instance...
I have just been to Prague,
and when we got there my girlfriend,
obviously, she likes to do the cultural thing,
so if they have a meal that they're renowned for something, or a dish or something...
she would really like to sample that,
and what I find is
that when I'm dealing with ..
because there were so many other new things which I was dealing with,
new territory, not knowing where I was,
my dependency had gone through the roof on every level,
I can't cope with trying or doing anything new,

Sue: when you're already doing everything new..

Yes,
and I'm already dependent,
I just need something that is familiar,

That I'm anchored again in some way,
and so I'm starting to realise
that whenever other people are wanting to do new
and try new things,
it is always when I'm feeling resistant to do it,
and I've always thought;
what the hell is the matter with me,

I've always thought that ...I've got some sort of reactive mental problem
because, when everybody wants to do something new
because the opportunity is there,
I can't embrace it.

And I'm really starting to realise now
that it always coincides,
my resistance always coincides with when there is lots of change
and my dependency has gone up.
Because another time...

Sue: If you were feeling..
confident, safe, secure....

You would be quite happy to do that new thing.
But when you've got everything..
like going to a new country,
where you know where everything is different and you're dependent
for everything ....

Everything.
And I can't ...
it doesn't feel safe for me to try something even like
a new spread on a piece of bread.
It sounds crazy, but it's so real
and I guess that lots of people use food as a form of addressing
some kind of
control issue,
and that's how it works for me.

Sometimes you just want something
that you know what it's going to feel like,
what its going to taste like
and what its going to do to your body,
and that might be just a dry bit of bread,
and that's what creates a secure anchor
in somebody who is experiencing such dependency.

The other issues that I find as regards control is;
again being by myself I don't experience this,
when I'm not in an intimate relationship with somebody,
so I'm not **feeling** to the same level,
then I don't experience this,
but when I am,
I really struggle with my partner using some kind of mind altering substance,
whether it be alcohol or drugs, or even prescriptive medication
because they all come under a similar umbrella.

Sue: they all affect...

and compromise somebody's ability to …
when you are at somebody's mercy
and you are dependent
then it just does not feel safe
or natural
for somebody to compromise that..

Sue: Because they're not just compromising their safety,
and how they are, they are compromising how much …
where you are
and how you're feeling.

And so this is something in relationship
which I've so struggled with,
I cannot tell you how much I've struggled with it
and there are times when I just …
when I would just so love to be able to drive
so that I can set myself free,
and I could ..

Sue: Driving is huge isn't it,
really?

Yes.

So I do feel that my partner,
she is not as free as she could be because I'm saying to her, "look
you know there are times when I'm ok about you drinking two or
three glasses of wine, but there other times
when I can't cope with that, it instils so much anxiety in me"
that….
I find that so difficult,
and yet I know, this isn't exclusive to me
because there are other people who feel like that,
but I also know loads of other blind people that get drunk
themselves,
and love drinking,
and have no issues being around other people…
I don't know,

I think I've developed a few physiological receptors for fear of
alcohol,
but,
I do find though that it's not conducive for me to be at the mercy of
somebody who's
not in control,
or not feeling the same,
or you know…

I know that people might say,
"how would you deal with going to a party if you're blind and you're
not in a relationship and there's other people drinking?"

The thing is that quite often you haven't got to go to that party,
it's not that you've got to go
because your girlfriend wants you to go….

Sue: And if you're going independently,
you would go knowing what ….
If I'm going somewhere like that
on my own,
I plan it meticulously,
I know how I'm getting there,
I know how I'm getting back,
I know where the loos are,
I know how...

It's much more prescriptive isn't it?

Sue: But when you're in a relationship and go with somebody else
and they're taking some of that responsibility
then it's really hard isn't it?

Yes definitely.

Sue: Because they're wanting to go...
and not always wanting to think about you all the time.
No.

So…identity,
control,
authenticity,
power ….

Since my research activities started I have really begun to
appreciate that what I see of the world is very different to what
other people see (both physically and metaphorically). A few weeks
ago I stood on one of the hills that surround my home with a friend
and asked her what she could see, and what that told her about
herself. Her response was very interesting.

"I can see what seems like the whole of Wales set out before me, the
hills, the valleys, and the beautiful sky. It reminds me of how much I
belong to the earth, and how the city in which I live consumes me
and turns me into someone I don't want to be. I also feel sad that
you may not be able to see this view and share this moment with
me."

Unsurprisingly my view was different. I could only see one tree,
the leaves shining in the summer sun. What was more important
however was that I could feel the wind in my hair, the sun on my
face and smell the mixture of sheep and wet grass. I was on a path
I knew and felt comfortable with. I felt vitally alive and happy.

Which view represents the truth I wonder? What became the truth was when we started to talk to each other about what we could see and its' meaning for us, what emerged was something different. My friend was able to understand my viewpoint, and I hers, and this mutual understanding became the reality for us. Truth was not just visual, but more a social process that included the visual, but also included listening to each other and feeling the wind in our hair. She no longer felt "sad" about something she assumed was important to me, and I understood more about what the visual meant for her.

People so often make assumptions about what people who are visually impaired might think, feel, need based on their own commitment to vision and what is important. Perhaps instead of making assumptions it would be better to have a dialogue that does not always assume that "sighted" is always better!

CHAPTER SEVEN

WHO AM I IF I CANNOT SEE YOU?

This chapter explores identity issues related to gender, sexuality and relationships with sighted people and includes part two of the commentary entitled: "re-authoring blindness"

Journal 19 October 2008
Who am I?
Do I define myself in not seeing what's not there?
Why should I? It's just not there.

Still within, the child who dreams of being a ballet dancer,
twisting and twirling round the kitchen floor,
weaving stories of magic and pixies in the woods.
I find myself here.
Also, when I walk in the hills,
feel the sun on my face,
the rain in my hair,
see the view that takes my breath away.

I find myself when I talk to you, feel the spark, the connection that links us, the passion, the pain, the laughter, the tears.

I find myself through my love of others, and their love for me.
I find myself in the kitchen, baking a cake, cooking a meal.

I find myself in the quiet still of God.

But not, never in the bit of vision that is missing.
If it is missing, and never has been part of me,
how can absence be defining?

I am defined sometimes by the things this lack of sight makes more difficult,
the mobility,
accessibility,
that it takes me so much longer,
and so much more effort to do the same tasks.

I am defined sometimes by what other people say,

or don't say, about my lack of sight,
the words that take something away,
something more important than the sight that isn't.
Words like,
"useless"
"stupid"
uttered by those not understanding my lack of sight,
they stay with me,
unwelcome guests,
and become part of who I am.

Or, the pitying patronising words
of those who think they understand my vision,
but don't.
And my anger at that.

I am defined by my friendship and comradeship with other visually
impaired people,
and rejoice and relax,
that I never have to explain.

By my family,.
who always treat me like a "normal" person,
and accept me for who I am.

Re-authoring Blindness (Part Two)

It is a myth that people who are blind or partially sighted have compensatory heightened other senses, such as hearing, touch, or smell (RNIB 2008) but, I think that I have learnt to use other senses in order for me to make sense of my life. Although I have relatively good forward vision, my responses to both my inner world and my relationships with others are usually in terms of the kinaesthetic, rather than the aesthetic, in other words, I tend to assimilate knowledge through "feeling" rather than "sight". I use sight as well, but this is usually secondary to the "feeling" response. When I use the kinaesthetic sense, the responses I have are embodied, for example, as you talk to me although I may be listening carefully, and seeing you in part, my body resonates with the timbre of your voice, the emphasis you put on certain words, my breathing falls in line with yours. I am aware of my own inner world, and the difference speaking to you makes to me, and the possible impact I am having on you. Being aware of and analysing these responses I am then able to translate them into thoughts, words and behaviours. These are skills that I have always used intuitively, and honed such that they are helpful to me in my work as a counsellor. And they are indeed helpful when working intimately with one or two people but, if I need to connect with a crowd of people, for example presenting a paper at a conference, or talking to group of friends in a pub, or negotiating my way through a crowd of people, then these embodied responses are not quite so helpful, because I cannot pick up on them in the same way. I am too far away, people are not talking to me directly, and there are just too many people.

It is often in these situations that my sight is also at its weakest. If I am sitting in a chair opposite you and having a private conversation, providing the lighting was good, I would be able to see part of your face, and have time to pick up images about your body language and what you might be wearing. If however I am sitting or standing at a distance where there are many people gathered, even if the lighting is good, I cannot see more than fleeting confusing images, and I am not always able to pick up the clues that I need to feel connected to the group, or even find my way through a busy train station. At these times I feel disconnected and fragmented, and often afraid.

I like to think that visual impairment has not impacted on my sense of self as a woman, or on my sexuality and relationships, but deep down I sense that if I was sighted it would be different. Perhaps I would not have the love for wearing bright vibrant colours – pastel shades do not register anything other than grey. Perhaps my relationships would be different if they were based on what I can see rather than what I feel and hear of the other.

Although I am very good at exploring my relationship with my inner world, and what this means to me, and the relationships I have with individuals, I find it much more difficult to examine my relationship with larger groups in the outside world. It takes longer for me to assimilate the information, and often I do this from a position of vulnerability (because of feeling disconnected and fragmented), and often if people are aware of my visual impairment then it also includes their pre-judgments about what this may mean; assumptions are made which are often inaccurate.

It has helped me to consider that I can define myself through the stories that I tell of these inner and outside relationships, rather than accepting that they are fixed, and intrinsic to my personality. If they are stories, then I can re-negotiate, or as White says "re-author" (White 1995) them. I can change or re-author the story I tell of feeling "disconnected from people" because of my visual difficulties, to being "differently connected to people". This gives me choices about whether or not to be transparent about both my visual difficulties and my thoughts and feelings in the moment. For example, at the beginning of a presentation instead of feeling disconnected, but feeling unable to do anything about this, I can talk directly to the audience about how difficult it is to make a connection with them without sight, this then changes my experience from feeling disconnected to feeling that even if they are sleeping, and disinterested I, at least, have stepped towards them, and offered an invitation to conversation. If the presentation is about blindness I have sometimes invited audiences to listen to the presentation without looking at the power point, and this has provoked much interesting discussion and made connections in ways that before would not have been possible.

Within social settings it is more difficult and challenging, because in articulating my feelings and needs I am setting myself apart from the group, and changing the dynamics in ways that I may not wish (do I always want to be the centre of attention?) and possibly overshadowing the differing needs of others, and I am also interacting with people who may have very set ideas on what a visual impairment means and may not be at all interested.

One very inspired person (who would like to remain anonymous) I worked with last year, taught me that you cannot always change the public's reaction to blindness, but that you can change how you react to their words and actions. She discovered that if instead of interpreting the sighted person and their insensitive comments as "insulting" she re-defined them as "disabled in understanding", she could then have more "patience with them, because of their disability", and then felt "less hurt and angry" and that this had made her daily life "more tolerable", as she told me, "I get these sort of comments all the time, and I can't let them get me down" (included with permission).

Andy notices the differences as he moves from a sighted world to a non sighted one. He tells me that for him his sense of self as a man, and indeed his sexuality is "a very visual thing" and now he has to change to him being more reliant on his sense of touch, but within what he describes as "polite society" this is not always possible, then he feels unsure about who he is.

Andy: Who am I as a man anyway?

I run my hands over my body,
my fingertips can explore and know these things.
The stubble on my chin.
The chest hair.

But am I a man to you?
I hear your voice
I catch a smell of something feminine

A glimpse of orange – skirt I think
But I can't see your face.

I can't touch your body.
I have to follow the etiquette of the sighted.
If I could see I would see in seconds what it takes me for ever to tell.

I can only be a man if I can gauge myself against you as a woman or perhaps someone else as a man.

I took it for granted when I could see. Constantly taking in what you look like and the differences between us.

This leads me to know who I am, and who you are, and whether we can be together or share any level of intimacy.

So alone. That is my experience of blindness.
So alone.
So not knowing.

Sometimes being alone.
Knowing it will always be like this..
I want to die.
Don't want to go on.
Living isn't something I do at the moment.
This is just survival stuff.
The aloneness.
Set apart – just a thing.
Sexless.
Knowing-less.

My body constantly tenses against the emptiness.
Awaiting I know not what.
Set apart unless someone chooses to approach me.
Then there is no warning.
I don't see them coming – or going for that matter!
I get no choices about who I talk to.

For me to know intimacy now there has to be touch.
If I touch your hand I suddenly see – your face, your heart, your meanings,
or try to.

You understand I think.
Your hand pulses with life.
I have met you,
your hand is a window,
A moment of meeting.

Adam also talks further about his experience of losing sight and how it affects his relationships with others:

Adam: But the problem is that sight loss
is such an active acutely active; 24 hours a day thing
It's not a passive experience,
it's such an active experience.

Sue: because it affects everything? ..

Every single moment.

I think as regards "relationship",
Whether that be with your telly,
or other people,
or just the world; society in general

I think a wonderful example of that
    and I think I know you understand this one,
is walking by yourself with sight loss;
is so different to walking in relationship with somebody else.
On the same pavement.

It is so much more difficult, unless you join.
But when you join,
then you enter a different relationship..

Sue: and you lose something?
Or you gain something?

Well I think it is a paradox..
well I think everything about sight loss is a paradox,
I think it is both.
It's both.

But as regard to my masculinity I do really struggle
with...
I don't when I'm on my own....

I don't when I'm on my own
it feels very different in relationship
there's something about
being in a relationship which really mirrors that.

Sue: Any relationships?

I suppose I can only speak for myself,
but an intimate relationship with a woman,
my experience with being with other men
is kind of like as friends
is different again,

it's different again,

I don't seem to have the same desire

or need
to be a man with another man,
so it doesn't hook the same things in me.

Sue: And has that got easier over the years?

No I think it is getting harder,
because I'm losing more sight,
and I'm more aware,
I think ...
If you think of a triangle;
and you put over the top of a triangle power,
and each point is a different aspect of power,
you've got individual power,
role power,
cultural power,
I think I'm very conscious
that there's times when I move into areas of strength
regarding power,
such as;
at times I move into quite strong role power,
there's times when my individual power is very weak,
and there's time when it is very strong,
and I know that we all experience
these shifts of power in those domains.
But it can happen in a split second ..

You can be so vulnerable
and so dependent
and the changeover can be a second...
it's incredible.
Just so fast.

Sue: So noticing that..
does that help you address those moments when you feel as though
you've lost power?

Well I'm very conscious of what's going on
and feel very grateful that
I am
kind of aware,
but I don't think
that awareness....

There's a price to pay.

It can be very exhausting.
Very exhausting.

The whole journey all my life
as regards my sight loss
has **absolutely**

put me inside.

The relationship I have with my internal world is ...
increasing,
and is already very, very, very strong.
It is increasing,
and for that reason alone
I feel very blessed.

And I feel blessed,
because I feel like I am blessed,
and it is a wonderful...

it has been a wonderful teacher
and a wonderful opportunity,

but what did happen to me in psychotherapy
is...
I think
I was using the blessing,
and the silver lining,
and the teaching of the experience of sight loss
as a survival mechanism
to avoid some of the more frustrating....

Well I actually discovered
that I didn't feel very free to be frustrated and angry
because, the way that I operated
and the condition of worth that I had put on me by everybody else
was;
I was "Mr Cope"
Mr "Coper"
and fantastic at dealing with it,
and I was not free to feel the other things
which naturally are part of the process.

Adam: So that was actually a real tough thing for me.

Sue: Sounds as if it was quite liberating though?

Yes.
Yes, very liberating
it set me free.
It did set me free,
but very difficult,
very difficult process.

Working as a counsellor I am often in conversation with people of
older years who were losing sight through macular degeneration, or
glaucoma. Often women talk to me about how sight loss leaves

them with a sense of loss and a "not knowing" who they are any more. Mo sends me a poem following the end of our counselling sessions and asks that I use it within my writing. She speaks of her visual image that has become familiar with the passing of years, and what it is like not to be able to either see that image or present it to others.

The mirror tells lies.

Coral lipstick,
aqua shadow
brown eyeliner
mahogany tint

my public face for so long

The mirror tells lies now
the lips misaligned
gaping cracks indeterminate.

no lips,
no shadow,
no tint

A grey ghost
Who is it?
Not a woman,
an "it".

Annie also talks to me about how not having so much control over her appearance affects her:

Annie: It is silly really..
It really matters to me to put on my lipstick.
That sounds very vain and stupid I know,
but somehow it gives me confidence.

Sue: It gives you confidence to be you?

Yes. that's it.
That's it. I can be me.
Now when I look in the mirror I can't see my lips unless I sort of squint sideways.
I was so frustrated that I would sit on the edge of the bath and sob, but the girl who comes to help me with mobility said she thought that I had put it on for so long I would probably be able to do it with my eyes closed..
and I could,
just by feel, and she told me when I had it looks fine.
So that's what I do now.
I put it on with my eyes closed.

It seems silly for an old woman like me to be worried about my looks,
but I'm not sure that it's about what I look like,
I think it is more about what I feel like inside,
and all the things I have lost.
I need something that anchors me to who I am,
and that others will recognise that it's the same person inside.

Sue: I'm wondering what it is about that "you inside" that is important?

I suppose it is about strength,
I have survived a lot of things in life,
had a lot of joy and a lot of sadness,
Have been a wife, attractive and loved,
and then lost.... and grieved.
But those things made me stronger,
made me into a woman, a proper woman.
I don't want to lose sight of those things.
Wearing lipstick,
finding a new way of doing it,
reminds me of those things and links me to ideas that are
bigger than the blindness.

Will emails me after reading Dennis, Adam, Tony and Mike's stories:

Hi Sue,
I can't tell you how important it feels for me that blind people have a voice and try to explain to the outside world how our lives are.

You asked me how these stories resonated with my own experiences.

The feelings of being a fraud, because I have some residual vision, and people sometimes seeming as though they are trying to catch me out. The anger at finding it so hard to get proper employment which has dogged me for ever, and the assumptions that other people make about my life and needs, and as I have said to you before the fact that I was never allowed to say that I did not like or want to be blind. I grew up in a family where I had to be well-adjusted and not upset my parents.

I suppose the stories that resonated for me most were Mike and Adam's, especially Adam's – I also have RP and when Adam was talking about his relationships and how difficult it is to remain authentic when affected by a degenerative condition, where how you are now could be different next week I thought I wanted to ring him up and say "yes. Yes".

I think sight loss has affected everything about me as a man. There is something masculine about "being the breadwinner", and "taking care of" the woman, which I can't do, not for want of trying I might add. I know in this age of equal opportunities it is not something I should say, and probably should not matter, but to me it does and affects my sense of self.

Not seeing also affects my sexuality, which I realise is a very visual thing even if I only have a little residual vision. Even the ability to get started with a relationship (other than friendship) is much more difficult. I can't tell whether she is attractive to me or not – you can hardly go over to what you think might be a woman standing at the bar and run your hands across her contours!! Sorry. Probably too much information!

I wrote this poem in my journal recently, thought you might be interested:

<blockquote>

They think they understand,
but it is like trying to travel to a different culture.
Different world.

You can step in my shoes for a moment,
but later you can
get back in your car,
drive home
switch on the TV.

Being blind is being invisible.
It doesn't just take your ability to see,
but either,
sticks you out like a sore thumb
or leaves you mindless, opinion-less
and grateful.

So grateful all the time.
People expect it.

I pretend sometimes I can see
going down town.
The simple pleasure of pulling it off without being caught,
or humiliating myself by falling over a trash can.
As a teenager I believed that no-one would ever want me.
My sexuality felt different.
My brothers talked of seeing a woman's leg, her breasts,
pawing through secret stacks of
girly-mags.
I wondered and hated not seeing.
The awfulness of not knowing,
the outsider.

</blockquote>

Yet inside,
I sensed women as being different,

I remember being about 15
going with my brothers to a club.
The girls hung around us.
There was something cool about them hanging out with the blind guy!
It was after all the era of the musical "Tommy".
Sitting on my knee,
making faces at each other.
Twittering like birds,
scented of sunshine and lycra.
Then as the evening went on
people paired off.
Danced.
I was left alone,
minding,
but unable to move,
go home.
Waiting.
Hoping they would remember me.

Other times, I was seen as a friend,
a "safe" brother
almost asexual.

"I like you" Cindy said
"but not in that way".

I wondered about my face.
Were my spots worse than other peoples?
Was my hair different?
Was I wearing the right jeans.

I met Jo when I was about 38
I thought that I was destined to being celibate.
I yearned for a family.

My daughter is now 21 and planning on getting married.

I saw her born – thank God,
but I will not be able to see her get married.

CHAPTER EIGHT

BLINDNESS AND DISABILITY DISCRIMINATION

In earlier chapters contributors talk about how their interactions with others have affected their sense of self within this chapter this theme is expanded to include an exploration of how disabling practices have disempowered or in some cases empowered contributors. There is also part three of the commentary entitled re-authoring blindness.

Journal: 27th November 2008

Lying in the bath, I allow myself to sink down under the water.
I feel the warm pressure against my eyes,
a sense of freedom,
escape.

I want to give up.
I want it to stop.

I feel so overwhelmed by the feelings I have about the research at the moment.
    "Bambalela,
    Bambalela,
    Oh
    Bambalela,
    Bamba, Bamba, Bamba Bamba
    Oh
    Bamba- le- la

    Never give up,
    never give up,
    Oh..
    Never give up,
    never, never, never,
    never,
    Oh..
    Never, never give up"

Music from Iona written by a struggling church in South Africa wafts
up through the floorboards and touches me in the bath.
I surface,
tears run down my face.

No I will not give up,
but I am overwhelmed for a moment by my emotional reaction to
the research.

I am immersed.
This is not a process where I am an independent observer,
nor is it a professional relationship,
like a counselling relationship.

This is about me,
about others,

I feel their emotion,
I feel my own,
anger,
sadness,
fury at
unfairness,
judgement
and for everything being such hard work.

I am afraid that all of this will be meaningless.
I have sent the stories I have so far out to a group of people who
have agreed to be witnesses to our stories.

I wait in the silence for a response.

As more people speak to me about their experiences of being visually impaired I am overwhelmed, not just by the research process, but also by anger at the injustice and unfairness people face as they try to go about their normal lives. Within medical, social and employment settings people are "disabled" by the practices of the majority (who are sighted). I am also afraid that the stories so painfully told will be devalued or dismissed by people reading them. This fear is born out of personal experience where my own views as a visually impaired person have been discounted. I am after all the one with the problem, the one who is lacking vision.

Disabling Practices

What are disabling practices? These could be seen practices that exclude disabled people from everyday activities, such as accessing education, transport or even employment and leisure activities. Governments over the last couple of decades have responded to pressure emanating from disability groups and worked to promote more inclusive practices. For visually impaired people this has meant more crossings with tactile cones that vibrate when it is safe to cross, clearly marked crossing points with tactile floor coverings, information available in a variety of mediums, "access to work" initiatives that have enabled many visually impaired people to access employment.

There is however another kind of disabling practice that is inherent in our society, even within those organisations specifically set up to support people who have disability, and this is located within the attitude that we have about disability, especially blindness. As we have seen in previous chapters those who are blind are often thought of either in terms of pity or they are seen as some kind of "super-hero" valiantly battling though life with their guide dog or white cane. Contributors have often found sighted others making assumptions about need and of discounting what the person living with a visual impairment is saying. It is as if their voice is unimportant set against professional and public opinion. The person has to manage both their own thoughts and feelings regarding their visual impairment, and also the responses of the world around them. As Mintz points out impairment itself is "both a lived experience and an effect of discourse" (Mintz 2007:3). Tuttle and Tuttle describe the experience of blindness as:

> "both a physical and psychosocial phenomenon. The medical component provides data regarding etiology, diagnosis, prescription, and prognosis. However, it is more important that the experience of living with a severe visual impairment be described in terms of the interaction among three elements: the needs and desires of an individual with little or no vision; the physical and social environment of that individual; and the common perception of blindness" (Tuttle and Tuttle 2004:5).

It would seem that all three of these elements can have an effect on how people feel about their visual impairment, and the latter two; the social environment and common perceptions of blindness have a huge impact on both self esteem and identity claims.

One of the themes that re-occur most frequently in the conversations I have had with people who are visually impaired over the years is their interaction with organisations who claim that they have non-discriminatory practices, but often in practice are not able to offer more than token support to those with different needs.

Tony copes well with reduced vision but talks of his frustration at never having his ideas or needs taken into account. He feels (as do others I have talked with) that often "lip service" is paid to disability discrimination, and often policies are "words rather than actions". Discrimination he considers is less overt – "people do not say we will not employ you because you have a disability, they use a different excuse, but there is still no job!" (Tony). He often feels although technically as a "service user" his opinion is asked for, it is never listened to or taken seriously.

Within this excerpt of conversation we talk here about ongoing battle with his local eye hospital where he has been asking them for nearly two years to send him appointments in large print:

Sue: I've always sensed that there is a lot of frustration, for you, because you have lots of ideas, and do your bit..
but other people don't always respond.

Tony: I'm basically an ideas person as you've found out, possibly my difficulty is getting the ideas across, or finding a channel for the ideas.

Sue: It's finding that channel isn't it, and other people facilitating that...

Take the eye hospital,
My achievements with the organisation that tries to represent patients
has been very little, because they haven't brought in anything yet.

Sue: Do they still send you small print appointments?

Oh yes.
I want large print,
this is the size of the print,
which I think you've seen,

" Bristol Eye Hospital appointment time"

I can't see it other than if I bear down very uncomfortably with a magnifier..

There is no..
they might be wonderful surgeons there,
    but even they don't have much power..
They should be able to say this is unacceptable for people.
But why don't they **do anything**?
I mean it's not a big deal is it?
Is it a big deal to get large print?

Sue: For an eye hospital? No. I think it would be fundamental!

I think that is where the RNIB,
and they might have been talking for years and years,
but they want to step up their action about it.
As I said at the advisory meeting, it's no good having a toothless …
It's got to **do something**,
If it doesn't do anything constructive…
there is no good having play meeting sessions,
you want something that's going to bring about change.

If I don't see change,
then I get
very frustrated and bored by it all.

Sue: Yes. Yes. Because you think "what is the point?"

What is the point?
Yes.
Exactly.

You're wasting your breath,
you're just saying "oh yes",
and they nod their heads.

Sue: But unless something actually happens…
It's a big organisation..
my concern is that it's a large organisation
they've got a lot of power over people's lives.
Why don't they use it?

This is what we've discussed before;
the way power is used.
Why don't they use it?
In a positive way.

Sue: And the frustration is that you can go and say all these things at meetings, you can talk to PAL[1] and you're still getting appointments in small….

I mean they probably mean well,
they'd love to be able to do it
but they don't pull..
I nearly said pull their finger out..
but that's probably the right word isn't it?

This is a general point by the way, not an individual's.
A general point that "they" don't like rocking the boat.
If they've got the boat ..(shows rocking motion)

Sue: Just a gentle swish..

─────────────────

[1] Patient Assistance and Liaison

You mustn't make waves!

Sue: 'cause what would happen if they made waves?

Probably it would be too dangerous (almost a whisper)
It would be too dangerous.

Sue: Someone might fall out?
(laughter)

Well we all fall out at times,
I've certainly fallen out in my time, many times.

Sue: But that kind of attitude is so difficult.

I've come across it all the time.
All my life with, one thing and another
I've come across;
   brick walls,
   fences,
   hurdles,
   many of them I've been able to clamber,
   over,
but a lot of them I haven't been able to clamber over.
That's where the mixture of;
   frustration and impotence,
   and **sheer,**
     sheer,
   dark depression
has come in.

You can't shift them.
They're so set in their ways,
I am set in my ways..
but not when it comes to ideas.

Thousands of people go to the eye hospital every year,
they've probably got worse eyesight than I have!
And I've got very poor sight.

Sue: How about the privacy,
if you get something you can't read,
it means that somebody else has got to read it...

It's a problem,
I don't want to ask others...

It's about privacy,
other people reading my mail,
when it could be personal,
or just...

my mail just piles up.
Unless it is in very large print and then I read it with difficulty.
I mean I've got some eyesight,
but not enough to read with comfort.
And there are not many organisations deal with that request for large print ..
They think that large print is "this"..
According to the eye hospital, this is supposed to be their largest font
or whatever it is called...

Sue: ..Well I can't read that...

I couldn't see that number

if you picked me up and glued me on there.
Glued the paper to my eye..
but I just think that it's so topsy-turvy
in their quest for numbers games ..

Sue: It's been a lifetime of frustration..

I go round trying not to look frustrated,
I mean my friend (name deleted) said yesterday,
  "you know Tony...
  the reason I like you...
  is because....
  of what you've been through....
  and how you try to cope with it..."

I very rarely talk about my own situation unless I'm with you,
or someone who I know very well;
which is few and far between.

Even those I know very well....

Sue: But she sees that,
and that's why that's very precious.
She sees some of the things you've been through,
and how you try and cope with it...

And in my peculiar way,
I do try and cope with it.

If I'm feeling miserable,
I am not miserable out there,
I'm more miserable in here.
You know sort of
that's when my ..
  I'm going round in a circle sometimes,
but I try not to be miserable when I'm talking to other people.
I might say I'm not brilliant today,
but that's about as far as it will go.

But I wouldn't say that even, very often.

A mask.
You've got to wear a mask.
Otherwise if I was ..

You don't always want people you don't know
to know how you feel, do you?

That's why I've only been to the Samaritans twice in my life.
While they do a good service to a lot of people,
for me you are talking to strangers you might not see again.

But of course they haven't got the answer to your problems,
they're a listening post, like you are.
But you are a listening post in a different way.
You're a person.
Not post.
You know what I mean!

Sue: In some ways because all of us have different personalities....

We've all got personality disorders in some way or other
or difficulties..
I use the word difficulties.
    None of us are A1 are we?

We've all got our quirks,
big Quirks, small quirks ...you name it.

Emma emails me in response to a conference presentation by
Tony and myself:

Hi Sue,
I think that the way society thinks and treats people who are
different (people like me) really stinks. Even when you are little
you're always taught from a sighted perspective. It's always rammed
down your throat that you are different and that you need to fit in.
You're expected to either minimise the effect not seeing has on your
life and be grateful and polite to those around you. Everything is set
up for the sighted with occasional (when they feel like it) concessions
for those who don't see, and when things are offered it's like they're
giving you the crown jewels!

I've always hated having to use a white cane, and that my eyes look
funny. Years ago I was advised to wear dark glasses so that my
appearance didn't "upset" other people. Why the f*** should I? I
was sent off for anger management once when I was at school, but
actually I think that the anger is justified and is what keeps me sane.
If I give in and become "a good little blind girl" then I will lose
everything, my self respect, who I am, any sort of worth. The whole

question of discrimination is talked about now as if it is a matter of pretending people are not different. **But they are!** On the surface everyone is politically correct but underneath the sighted think that they are better than those who don't see. Some folks treat me normally, for which I am very grateful, but they are usually people who know me well and do not make assumptions.

Mo talks also about attitudes within social services and how these effectively "disable" her:

Mo: The first time she visited she brought me a talking watch and a white cane.
Which was very nice of her[2].
She kind of talked to me like I was a five year old though.
As if losing my sight had somehow left me with no opinion.

Sue: So the cane and the watch were helpful, but her attitude was not?

Yes, well, no
Actually I didn't want to use the cane. I said so,
she said that was very selfish of me,
I needed to consider other people, like drivers.

I remember thinking – Oh well perhaps I'll have to use it
But I didn't….

Everyone uses patronising voices
says "you mustn't let it get you down"
"think of all the things you can do"
I do know this,
but it's the patronising bit I can't stand
and no-one really gets that at all.
They think they are being really politically correct,
offering me large print letters and a cane
and expect me to be grateful.

Even within the organisations who have set themselves up to support people who are visually impaired there is often an attitude of "doing good for the poor blind people" (quoted verbatim from a potential volunteers application form). Having said this there are also many who work tirelessly with these organisations in hope of changing this attitude.

Mike talks about his experience of working for a leading charity supporting people who are visually impaired:

---

[2] Social Worker

Mike: I've taken an interesting journey,
impairment related journey, while I've been working for (name deleted)
(laughter)
I suppose my masters degree and subsequent working with (name deleted),
I kind of meandered between the sort of;
fairly militant disability rights movement,
   never quite feeling like I fitted in,
and the sort of;
"we're here to help you because you have a visual impairment" world of the (name deleted).
Although I think that the organisation's moved quite a long way,
I'm not saying it's moved as far as I might like....

Sue: but it moves between those two spaces?

I find myself being the bridge...
A bridge which sometimes feels;
incredibly trampled,
between those with extreme views,
the disability rights, almost at one stage saying;
"it's not about impairment at all"

Sue: It's about society's attitude and working to change those attitudes. The other side being "we're here to help the poor blind people.."

Yes.
I started off by thinking..
Feeling..
I **ought to** subscribe fully to the rights movement,
and I think probably rather than being a polar thing,
it's more like a sphere of; what's relevant at any particular time.

Because at the end of the day,
we experience the world through our senses,
so we need to come to a point of balance,
where we feel able to interact with the world with our senses,
and so we can't ignore that.

I think one of the struggles that I have had in my work,
and in the way we approach things,
is that we talk a lot about, "fixing",
   even if we've not talking in the spiritual sense about healing,
we talk a lot about fixing...

Just thinking about..
We have a brilliant counselling service..
A good one if I may say so...
(laughter)
Which is fantastic,

but generally,
we only talk about people needing counselling,
or emotional support,
if they are broken...

I suppose what I am saying is that
we don't offer it to everybody,
we don't take it as almost an acceptance,
that whether somebody has
had a visual impairment for a long time,
or acquires it later on in life,
the likelihood is that they haven't been able to work through their
identity...

Sue: because they've had other people's..
Impositions of what blindness might mean?

And their own....

Sue: Yes you are right... the counselling service is portrayed as a
service for helping broken people. I'm thinking...
This bridge bit....it must be a bit uncomfortable at times

I think it is.
The analogy of the bridge only works so far,
because although I talk about feeling trampled,
I'm not sure that the bridge is actually acting as a free flow
between one sphere and the other.

It feels more like that people are standing on the bridge,
having a little look,
and not going all the way.

Sue: Is that because people can relate to you as someone who sees
both sides of the argument?

Yes I think so.
I think I'm changing,

For me there's something about..
I'm gradually beginning to learn something about grace,
what's the Christian understanding of grace,
which is not rights,
and is not charity.

Sue: So is it somewhere between? Or something different?

I think it's something different really,
because grace (from a Christian point of view)
is about a generous God,
a loving God,
that affirms us in who we are,

and who God is creating us to be,
and the rights language doesn't work,
because God owes us nothing,
in one sense.

The charity doesn't work,
Because charity leaves the identity unchanged.

Sue: There's also a power differential?

Yes.
Absolutely.

Charity is a classical Christian virtue as well,
but I think we've possibly misunderstood what it means.
Often in terms of the early to mid twentieth century
the version of charity, is that;
"we do good to you, and in turn that makes us feel virtuous".

But that's not a dialogue,
that's keeping the giver and the receiver in the same power
relationship.
Whereas I think grace is more of a conversation,
where the giver and receiver are in a relationship of transformation.

I've been doing a lot of background work on liberation theology.

*Sue: there's something about the word "liberation" which is similar to
transformation..*

Yes.
I think liberating ourselves from our own perceptions,
our own limitations, expectations of others,
all that kind of thing is quite important.
I think that some liberationists would certainly see the role of grace
within liberation theology.

Re-authoring Blindness (Part Three)

Do we have to remain stuck within this cycle of societal
misunderstanding and misinterpretation of what visual impairment
means to us? There is no simple answer to this because changing
societal attitudes could take generations of campaigning and
education. What we can we change however is how we respond to
these attitudes. We do not have to accept these misinterpretations
as our truth. We can change the stories we tell of our lives within
relationships that are important to us, and in this way can influence
how we identify ourselves.

This does not mean that if we are blind we can miraculously
"see", or that we can change other people's attitudes towards us

but, if we can change the relationship we have with the label "blind" or "visually impaired" and how we feel about it, it can enable us to feel differently and be much more able to challenge disabling practices. Certainly from my perspective this is more than a linguistic trick, but a felt reality. As discussed previously, we may not always be able to change other people's attitudes towards us, but we can change how we respond to those attitudes.

May was in her late eighties when I met her and had been diagnosed with Age related Macular Degeneration. She considered herself a "blind woman", but considered that this blindness had been "put on me by the doctors, they have labelled me with it, I even have a certificate to prove it.. and now **it is all that I am**"(May). Within this position she was unable to see any possibilities for her life, "this is not living, this is just enduring" were her words (Dale 2008, 2009). By separating her from the problem, [narrative therapists would call this "externalising the problem" (Morgan 2000)] and enabling her to re-negotiate the influence blindness had on her life, May was able to connect again with other parts of her life which were not blind, her history, her love of music, her relationship with her husband. She had not regained her vision, but her sense of self and identity now included more than "blind".[3]

My studies have encompassed both those recently affected by sight loss, and also those who had lived with a visual impairment most of their lives.

For those who had recently lost sight (and certainly the majority of those who accessed the RNIB counselling project during 2005-2008 were in this category (Dale 2008, 2009)), personal grief and loss were key issues, as were the practicalities of living with limited vision, but societal attitudes towards blindness and disabling practices did very much contribute to how each person perceived their recently acquired visual impairment, and did in fact make coping with grief and loss far more difficult. For many, the main issues were about their own feelings both about blindness (which may have been influenced by societal attitudes), and about the practicalities of living with limited vision and having to manage the challenges of mobility and accessing information. This time of transition, often came with sometimes overwhelming feelings of loss, despair and anger and loss of identity as a "sighted" person. Many could not imagine living in the world without sight. Sarah says:

---

[3] For a fuller description of my work with May see (Dale 2009) and also Chapter Twelve.

Sarah: Each night I pray that I won't wake up.
But I always do.
It's always the same just at that moment of waking.
Hope then despair.

Andy says:

Life isn't worth living.
But I live it because I'm too afraid not to.
I wish I didn't have to.

Most of the people I worked with (including Andy and Sarah) did come to a point where they could see life as worth living, even without sight, but they needed to find alternative ways of making sense of the world.

Andy: I now see differently
touch is very important
my world is now a tactile world
I feel my way across town
I notice things which were
before absent.
I smell the rain on new grass,
feel it against my face,
the orange blossom tree
thirty steps to the left
of the fourth drive after Maple street.

I feel the hands of my partner
the tiredness in her voice
Working 40 hours a week and
relying on my vision
these were all aspects of life missing.

It does not matter
whether I am a man or a non-being

when I feel I become me
and me exists and can commune with you.

My aloneness is around me still
Living in a different universe from you.
An alien,
alienated by your (by your I mean the world at large) reliance on the etiquette of the sighted.

Your alienation gives me time,
gives me space
for connecting spiritually to the whole of the rest of the universe

even if you are not aware of it or my existence.

I define myself as a "feeler"
someone who feels their way around and who feels
anger, rage, sadness, joy.
Feeling is being.
"I am" because I feel. (Dale 2006, 2008a)

Exploring the life experiences of people who have like myself lived with a visual impairment for many years I was surprised that there were similar themes emerging, although there was a movement away from the overwhelming initial responses to losing sight being at the fore. For many however there was still a deep conviction that societal attitudes and disabling practices had a profound influence on how lives were defined. I talk here with Tony about his feelings of being patronised:

Sue: It's that not having any control,
or, "say"

Tony: That's the story of my life really.
Although I've been 27, 37;
I may as well have been 16
in their eyes,
in some people's eyes.
Not everybody.

I won't say everybody.
Those who don't really know me...

It's impotence,
I feel impotent.

Even now,
I feel partly impotent being here ...
I mean as opposed to being...

Sue: What..
because it's sheltered housing?

Yes, but that's not really it..
I mean I've got a certain amount of freedom here.
I've got a lot of freedom here,
other than being called over the intercom in the morning.

All they do is buzz around the different chalets
or whatever they call them,
every morning.
But that is rather annoying
like, if you were at home
and being asked every day,
"are you alright?",
and in your state of

possible bleary eyed-ness..

Sue: you don't really want to be asked that first thing in the morning!

No you don't
actually.
I've been in ….
if you switch it off
then they come round to make sure..
but not always.

They'd wait until you were dead!

Getting back to the work...
My life,
most of my life, as you probably already know,
is doing voluntary work.
With big periods of unemployment,
lack of real work..
no..
no voluntary work is real work,
sometimes, the other work is not real.

Sue: You feel that some of the work is "we're putting this here for you so that it is provided". But it doesn't feel real?

That's why I would never suggest to anyone going to a day centre,
or an activity centre,
there are some of the most reactionary people running them.
I only know because I have visited them.
And did have a short period many years ago..
Morning I think it was,
and **it drove me bananas** …
"cup of tea love?".
"Teatime".
The trolley would come round with the tea.

I just think this is not just my story,
but other people's story,
who are connected by visual impairment..
or any other impairment.
If you've got more than one impairment,

you're **doubly** affected.

Sue: But even the voluntary sector..

That's got rather too
choosy now.
I'm all for police checks,
if necessary,

but they sent me voluntary lists
sometimes, from the volunteer centre
of jobs they think..

When I say "volunteers", my conception of volunteering is someone
who wants to do something for the sake of other people.

Not somebody who already can do it!
Someone who is willing to be trained to do it.
Most jobs I've had from the volunteer centre have been,
"must have experience"
they may as well pay someone for that!
(laughter)
Well I want something,
I don't mind asking for a bit of experience,
but I don't want to see;
"work in museum –
must have experience of being a museum director".
That's nonsensical!

What I noticed during the research process was that the linking
our lives together around common themes and talking about these
issues did seem to free us from these disabling practices, and did
change the stories we were telling about our lives. There was a
definite movement away from feeling "disabled" to feeling
"enabled", and in turn this invited us to re-author what blindness
and visual impairment meant to us as individuals and as a group.

As you read these accounts of our lives, both those of us who
have lived with a visual impairment for many years, and those who
are newly diagnosed, hopefully you will realise that **we are all
unique, and live rich full lives.** Our identities are so much more
than just our visual impairments, even if when you see one of us in
the street with a white cane you may think, "S/he is blind", or "s/he
is visually impaired". As Runyan and Jenkins say,

> "You can use any term you like, but it doesn't define me. In the end,
> it's my responsibility to ensure that the attributes by which I would
> prefer to be defined are more visible to you than my blindness"
> (Runyan and Jenkins 2001:14).

Our personal responses to our visual impairments are varied,
ambivalent at times, but certainly not overwhelmingly negative. Our
experiences are marked greatly by our interaction with a world that
prizes the visual above all other senses such that when we interact
with this world we can become "dependent" or "vulnerable" or even
"victims", and how we negotiate these relationships and the stories
we tell of our experience is, I believe, key to how we fundamentally
identify ourselves and challenges the taken for granted assumption

that "seeing, or not seeing, as the case may be, is a primary defining characteristic of who we are" (Kinash 2005:1).

CHAPTER NINE

NEW TREATMENTS:
"A STEP FORWARD FOR HUMANKIND"
OR NOT?

Within this chapter there is an exploration of whether visual impairment is always a medical condition that needs "treatment" or whether it is just a different way of being. It also includes part one of the commentary entitled "living in the twilight zone" that starts to explore some of the differences between partial sight and blindness.

Journal 25 October 2008
I received this email this morning which has got me thinking again about new treatment possibilities:

Dear Susan,
Thought you might be interested in attending this!

Featured event: 4 December 2008 - Feed Your Mind at Lunch Time: "Stemming Vision Loss with Stem Cells - Seeing is Believing"

Abstract:
The London Project to Cure Blindness aims to use human stem cells to prevent blindness, restore sight and improve quality of life in patients with Age-related Macular Degeneration (AMD) within five years from its initiation in 2007. Our goal is to replace cells lost by disease at the back of the eye with human stem cells that have been transformed into retinal pigment epithelium cells (the support cells) and photoreceptors. These cells will then be surgically implanted into a clinical population of AMD patients.

I am sure that this is a treatment that many affected by AMD will hail as miraculous. After all, many who are affected by macular disease are people who all their life have been sighted, and want to find a way of restoring this vision, and research of this kind is important and very valid. **But** *there is something about the group's name, "The London Project to Cure Blindness" that makes me feel decidedly uncomfortable. If their project is to "cure" blindness then does that imply that all of us who are visually impaired are medically damaged and in need of a cure?*

Rebecca Atkinson who is losing her sight due to Retinitis Pigmentosa writes of the new treatment possibilities, in this case of gene therapy:

"Hurrah, you cry. I must be thrilled. Actually I am a bit confused. It is easy to assume that all visually impaired people will be hammering down the doors should gene therapy prove successful. But to say this is to assume that a blind life is lesser and that all blind people really want to be sighted. They don't". (Atkinson 2007)

And yet, what would it mean not to carry on looking for treatment possibilities for conditions such as Macular disease? I feel confused. Perhaps there is a difference between "losing sight" and "living with reduced sight". **To me, "losing" implies bereavement, transition, grief, "living with" implies embracing, or being part of.**

Looking through Stephen Kuusisto's web site, (he writes profusely about the experience of blindness), I just loved the heading for his web page **"Planet of the blind - It is not as dark as you think".**

Also these lines from one of his poems, which really speaks to me of the kind of struggle I have with saying boldly, "I can choose how I identify myself in connection with blindness", and the deadening effect of feeling dependent and out of control as I struggle against a tide of sighted perceptions of the world.

"I went alone in the late October night
Towards a copse where the last sun
streamed through branches,
A caprice of twilight,
Walked with my head up,
Shoulders squared
Like any living person
Without a proper country
& who in turn
Hears the live one
And the dead ones
In the poor drums of his shoes" (Kuusisto 2008)

The last few years have brought about many advances in medical science, and this has had a disturbing effect on many of us who had assumed that there would be no possibilities other than to live as a visually impaired person. For some, especially those who have recently lost sight, there is a desire for restoration of sight. Mo talks of her experiences of hope for a cure:

Mo: Every time I see something on the news,
you know,

about "new cures for blindness"
my heart misses a beat and I think,
perhaps there is hope.
When I see the consultant however
he usually brings be down to earth.
My family used to send me newspaper cuttings and such like
but even they seem to have given up hope now
Sometimes I wonder whether I ought to give up my hope for a cure..

Sue: you wonder whether to give up your hope of a cure?
Yes.
Sometimes the hope of going back…
It stops me from living now,
I seem to be wasting months.. years even,
hoping for something that might not happen.

Sarah emails me with her thoughts:

Hi Sue,
Good to hear from you and learn about the book!

You asked me what I thought about the recent news article about new treatment possibilities and what my thoughts were.

It is quite strange, because I think if you had asked me the same question a year ago I would have had a different answer. When I was first diagnosed, the most important thing always was finding some kind of treatment or cure, and when they told me there was no treatment for my kind of macular disease I was devastated, couldn't believe it. I could not imagine a life without sight it seemed intolerable. Strangely, over the last year or so, things have changed for me. I'm not sure how I'd feel now if someone told me I could regain the vision I have lost and have some new treatment that was available. It seems odd saying this, but somehow the thought of change, and putting myself back into a position of "hoping", makes me very nervous. It's not that I don't miss my vision or find living without it problem free. It is still frustrating and aggravating! I think it is more about going back to a position of raised hopes only for them to be dashed again. I don't think I could stand losing hope all over again.

Annie also talks to me about treatment possibilities:

Annie: I'd sell my soul if I thought I didn't have to be blind,
It is the worst thing ever to happen to me
If I thought there was some treatment I could have
I would find a way of paying for it.
But there isn't so I'm stuck
Hope that "one day there might be a cure"
keeps me going back and back to the eye clinic.

I cannot bear to think of what will happen if they cannot
stop my sight from deteriorating.
They try all sorts of things,
injections, laser treatment,
nothing really makes much difference,
but I always keep hoping,
they keep telling me to come back,
so I do,
Before the appointment there is always hope;
perhaps this time they will be able to do something,
then afterwards disappointment,
then I wait for the next appointment.
I keep looking at all the articles about "cures for blindness"
I just can't let go of the hope that eventually it will be for me.

Andy emails me with his thoughts in response to the newspaper article:

> Hi Sue,
> When I got your email and sat down to reply I realised that things
> have changed a lot for me over the last couple of years. Twelve
> months ago I would have done anything to get treatment that
> would restore my vision, it occupied all of my waking thoughts,
> now, if someone offered me treatment that was guaranteed to work
> then I would probably say "yes". But it certainly is not something I
> am researching on the internet every day. I suppose I have finally
> accepted that this has happened and I just need to get on with life!
>
> Bet you never thought I would say that! I seem to remember
> ranting at you for hours about how I would never accept blindness.

I wonder what people who have been visually impaired for the
many years think, whether this differs from the views of those
recently diagnosed. Patrick emails me

> Hi Sue
> Thank you for sending me the article in newspaper about new
> treatment possibilities. I read it with great interest and it evoked
> quite strong feelings.
>
> I have always been really upset when people (usually with good
> intentions) tell me excitedly about new treatments being developed
> and that this might mean I will be able to live a "normal" life. I
> consider that I already live a normal life, and I really object to other
> people thinking that I need treating in some way. I am not ill, just
> different!
>
> Sorry about the rant! I totally agree with Rebecca[1] there is always
> the assumption that to be blind is to be defective in some way, and I

---

[1] This refers to newspaper article by Rebecca Atkinson in the Guardian
17.7.07.

would strongly argue that it is not, it is just being different. I am not sure that I would be a very good sighted person, I have however worked very hard to be a reasonably successful blind one! Having said all that; I do think that perhaps for some people who have always lived with sight and then lost it the thought of a "cure" may be very attractive. It's about choices, about not making assumptions though isn't it?

I also talk to Adam about his thoughts about new treatment possibilities:

Adam: As you might remember,
I was in psychotherapy for 2 or 3 years during my training,
but obviously that was under the umbrella of being
a compulsory aspect of my course,
    which did taint the therapy.
However last year out of my course …
2 years after,
I decided to re-access psychotherapy,
with a specific agenda,
which was;
to look at my sight loss
and possible sight intervention.
So,
restoration of sight,
because of the new things which are going on….
    and that was an amazing experience for me.
It was just so different actually;
first of all choosing to have therapy,
and setting the agenda,
and the work that I did there was completely around identity;
and how much of me,
how much of me is my disability,
and how much am I me….
and where am I operating from the majority of the time.

Am I operating from my RP,
or am I operating from something different,
and would I choose intervention if it was available,
and what aspect of me would choose it,
what aspect of me ….

It was just a very powerful therapy for 10/11 sessions I think
it was…
and …

through that journey I learnt..
I just learnt so much about
who I've become,
and who I am in different situations,
and how I use,
sometimes abuse,

sometimes try and hide my disability.

It's just incredible,
and the actual thought
of somebody finding an intervention
and taking that away,

felt like somebody removing a whole cultural ...
huge thing.

It was just a huge ...
but nevertheless at the end of my journey
I actually did feel so much freer to actually choose the intervention,
because, I realised that there was so much about me
that actually the RP might have exacerbated,
but I think was there anyway, and,
I realised that there was so much of me that wasn't my RP.

Mike also talks with me about his views on "sight loss prevention" the ongoing mantra which the RNIB and other visual impairment charities adopt to underpin their work.

Mike: The other quick thing I just wanted to touch on
is this whole thing of "sight loss prevention".
It's a simple message really
is...
That **of course**
people who have been sighted all their lives
should be given every opportunity to retain their sight,
   I'm sure that most people would want not to lose vision.
And I wouldn't.

I talk about healing and all that sort of thing,
in the sense if somebody could guarantee that I wouldn't lose any more sight,
that would be fantastic!
That in a sense that would be a healing I would want,

and possibly given the diversity of RP (retinitis pigmentosa) conditions,
maybe something I've experienced already,
because it certainly hasn't deteriorated at the rate that a lot of people do..
   I'm still trying to work that one out...

It's very difficult for me to say..
if we find some genetic formula that prevents
people from being born as visually impaired.
   I mean they are still born, but they don't have sight loss,
then I think it would be very selfish of me to say that shouldn't happen.

Because whereas I feel I have a certain amount of identity;
as somebody who has a visual impairment,
who am I to impose that on somebody who doesn't choose it.

Sue: or their parents don't choose it?

So that's why I prefer to talk about sight retention
because sight retention can apply to those not yet born,
it can apply to those of us who have a visual impairment
but they want it not to get any worse,
and it can apply to those who are sighted, and want to remain so.
For me... the trouble with sight loss prevention,
that it is a value statement
which disenfranchises those of us who have a visual impairment..

Sue: Yes. It makes us less than..

Absolutely..
And I know that there is a problem with the language,
because the language we live in ..
this unfortunate culture which where everything has to be marketable;
and sight loss prevention is a lot more marketable than sight retention...
and I think that's a problem..

Sue: sight retention is not the. "in phrase" is it?

And yet,
I don't think that a lot of people have even considered what
"preventing sight loss" means.
I think that for some they would say,
"of course you must prevent sight loss".
It seems to them obvious because it is a commonly held assumption.
It's only if you're standing at the side of the divide, if you like,
that "it's not ok to say that".

And at the end of the day I don't want to get caught up on linguistics, but it's the basis behind the attitude..

Sue: Well it is the attitude isn't it...that forms the language, and
it's the attitude that says.
however politically correct you are...
"if you're sighted you're ok, and if you're not then you are not".
And that kind of phrasing for me emphasises the feeling.
That you're ok if you have 20/20 vision, and if you haven't got 20/20 vision
you're on the other side of the divide.
But I don't know...
I think it's going to take quite a lot of energy to change organisations.

Talking with Mike really helps clarify my thinking. Perhaps it is not so much about whether research and treatment possibilities should be explored, but about changing the underpinning grand narrative (White and Epston 1990) that "sighted is normal and visual impairment is not normal" this would then as Mike says enable people to speak of "retaining vision" which validates both the experience of those seeking treatment possibilities, and also those who are visually impaired and likely to remain so.

Another question which I will try to address during the next chapter is about the differences in experiences between living with partial sight and blindness and the effect this has on identity. Within this chapter the discussion starts with part one of the commentary "Living in the twilight zone" and then explores if these differences have any relevance in respect of treatment possibilities.

Living in the Twilight Zone (Part One)

Am I blind? No. Am I sighted? No. I am one of the tens of thousands of people in the UK who are registered as sight impaired but have some residual vision. It is estimated that 49% of blind people, and 80% of partially sighted people can recognise a friend at arm's length (RNIB 2008).

As Schinazi says partial sight "has often been described as *neither fish nor fowl* phenomenon. Visual loss is many times perceived as an all or nothing occurrence" (Schinazi 2007:2), and as discussed previously, societal attitudes often mirrors this. I sometimes feel neither one thing, nor the other. For most of my adult life I have lived as a sighted person without the sight, as Kleege states:

> "looking sighted is so easy. For one thing, the sighted are not all that observant. And most blind people are better at appearing sighted than the sighted are at appearing blind" (Kleege 1999:19).

Hiding my inability to see, has however tempted me to disown that part of me which is visually impaired, and instead take on the label of "useless" because in a sighted world I cannot compete with those who have 20/20 vision, I am slower, cannot drive, clumsier, get lost, misread things. However hard I try I cannot keep up. Yet the blind world is also alien. I can and do use the vision that I have to make sense of the world, and I cannot imagine a life without seeing colour, or a spectacular sunset or mountain-view, or negotiating unknown territory with a cane alone.

One of the comments I heard most frequently from people who accessed the RNIB counselling service was, "I feel a fraud" or "I'm not really blind" (Dale 2008), and people who lost sight during their adult life who were left with some residual vision, seemed to find it more difficult to adjust to living with a visual impairment than some of the people I worked with who had lost all of their sight. Rosemary commented recently "I keep hoping that my eyes will get better, somehow if my sight had completely gone it would have been easier. I would have been upset of course, but would have had to get on with my life, as it is, I just can't let go of wanting to see properly again" (included with permission). DeLeo et al comments:

> "A strong discrepancy emerged between the patients with different clinical prognoses, that is, between those blind and those affected by partial sight loss. The psychopathological picture was worse for those with partial sight loss who displayed a more marked presence of depressed mood, anger, and hostility. Correction of gradually deteriorating sight seemed to pose greater problems than adaptation to total, definitive loss. Completely blind subjects probably had to cope with an irrefutable handicap, forcing them to accept their new social role and making them more malleable to rehabilitation techniques that, objectively, permitted better social adjustment." (De-Leo et al. 1999:340).

There seems to be marked differences in how people view the new treatment possibilities emerging. People who have been sighted and then have lost sight, especially those recently diagnosed, often only talk in terms of wanting a cure, seeing this as the only reasonable solution to their difficulties, but as time passes and they become adjusted to sight loss the emphasis changes.

Those who have lived with a degree of sight loss for longer have differing thoughts, some like Adam and Mike have thought through carefully what treatment possibilities might mean for them. There also seems to be a difference between those who (like me) have some residual vision and do not want to lose it, and those who are without any residual vision. I discuss this with Patrick:

Patrick: I suppose because I have only known blindness it is difficult to think what it would be like to see.
I don't really know what seeing is.

Sue: So "seeing" is not something you know about?

No. People have tried to explain it,
but my construction of what is visual may be totally different to the reality.
I guess it is something like hearing or feeling it gives people access to what is going on around them.
I have no memory of "seeing".
So if someone says to me
"would you like to see again"

It is something that is **totally meaningless**.

I just cannot imagine it.

It also makes me angry, because it says that they consider my experience of life to be less than theirs.

Sue: It feels that they are devaluing your life experience?.

Yes. Always.
Yet, perhaps there is also a weakness in me.
I've only started to think about this since contacting you
really…
I guess I feel that I live quite a comfortable life,
so perhaps I am afraid that changing it….
Would I be as successful?
Would I fail…..
and become just like everyone else?

There's something in me that likes being different.
My difference is part of who I am.
Perhaps it is just as terrifying for me to think of becoming sighted as it is for others to think of being blind?

Having said that I do think that they should continue to do research.
If I had the choice of whether I was sighted or blind I would choose blind.
If I had the choice for my child
I would choose sighted …

It is just such hard graft sometimes.
Sighted seems an easier option,
would give them more opportunities.

For me – I don't need treatment 'cause I'm not sick!
(laughter)

I gave a presentation recently to a group of ophthalmologists and eye care specialists[2]. I felt very nervous. Dennis and I were the only people with visual impairment present, all the others were professionals who spent their lives treating people like us, and were committed to eliminating blindness.

Despite the audience being warm and receptive, there was still an element of the professionally sighted humouring the experiences of the visually impaired, also of scientific quantitative research being superior to qualitative research that promoted personal stories. One

---

[2] Age Related Eye Disease Conference (in association with MA Healthcare 2009) Institute of Physics London.

consultant on listening to the personal accounts of Sarah and Andy and the findings from a research project conducted by VICTAR[3] (where people reported their negative attitudes of being diagnosed and registered) said "I don't believe this happens, I have worked in many hospitals and this has never happened".

It is commendable for the medical professions to work towards finding cures for blindness, but surely there is also room for considering that not everyone who has a visual impairment considers themselves in need of a cure. Treatment possibilities should give opportunity but not negate the life experiences of those who are different.

Journal 30 October 2008

Because I am so good at hiding the things I cannot see it becomes second nature and as someone said to me the other week, "it is not what I can see that is the problem...Now what I can't see, that's where the problem starts!!"

I borrowed some sim-specs[4] (they simulate various eye conditions) some time ago, and my friend peered through them.

"This is just awful" she said. "I just couldn't cope if it was me"

"This is how I see" I say proudly.

But, It's true I am proud of my sight, but it's not true that she can imagine what living with my sight is like, because I have lived with it all of my life and my brain has adapted brilliantly. For those who are used to 100% vision, they would really struggle to lose 70% of it! and now my friend mourns, and sympathises? which is crazy.

My sight isn't a problem for me. I love that I can sit here with my digital recorder and watch the autumn leaves out of the window. I love that I can see the expression on my daughter's face, as she opens a present or my husbands as he tells me about his day. The things I can't see, well they are just not there. Sometimes I wish for more; I suppose that's only human. I wish I could see the "whole picture". A whole face, instead of just the eyes, or the mouth or the nose. A whole tree instead of just a few leaves. A whole sunset instead of just the colour. But, on the whole, I am glad my vision is how it is.

---

[3] Visual Impairment research centre based at Birmingham University.
[4] these simulate various eye conditions.

One day I was asked whether I would seek "these amazing new treatments" no; for me it would be like changing from a woman to a man. But, is that being selfish? What would it be like for my family if I could drive again? If I could do the things that at present they have to do for me?

CHAPTER TEN

DIFFERENCES BETWEEN BLINDNESS AND PARTIAL SIGHT

This chapter explores the differences and similarities of the experiences of people who are visually impaired. Those who are blind, and those who have some residual vision.

Journal 12th December 2008
I had an interesting discussion with Caroline today. She is totally blind and has been so since she was a very small child. We were thinking about the kind of things that are similar issues we face in life due to being visually impaired and the things that are different.

Caroline had originally contacted me following publication of some of the stories from my studies. We then met to talk further about her life experiences. What follows is excerpts from our conversation:

Sue: I am wondering... ...I know that I have always been visually impaired, but I am not blind, I do have quite useful residual vision. What do you think the differences are for people who are blind and those who have a significant visual impairment, but have some residual vision?

Caroline: I guess from being around people who are both blind, and those who have some sight I have always found the blind people are more well adjusted..
That sounds very kind of very judgemental,
but somehow if you are completely blind,
and you know that this is it,
you have to get on with it.
You have to use the cane,
you can't ever hide the fact that you can't see.

That means you still get all the crap from people on trains and in the street,
you know the;
"poor you"
"what a shame"
"you are so wonderful to be able to get out and about"
But, there is never that lingering thought of trying to get by visually.
You just can't.

If the vision is not there at all you have to use other skills.
Or, develop other skills.

When I was at school, those who were blind were a kind of group
that stayed together and supported each other.
We were kind of bonded by not seeing at all,
We made fun of the "resid's[1]"
Excluded them often from activities we had got good at;
like using long cane and Braille
and walking about in the corridors in the dark!

It was much harder when I left school and had to interact with
sighted people all the time,
then I wished that I had some vision and could
"get" what they were talking about.

Adam also talks about his experience of attending a "blind"
college, this conversation took place in the context of a group
meeting where we had been discussing societal attitudes towards
blindness, and the feeling that we all belonged to a "visually
impaired club":

Adam: It's interesting
Dennis was talking about the "v.i. club".
I remember when I was at Hereford RNC for three years and I had
direct evidence there to the fact that there was also …
what we're talking about in society,
    this "us and them",
it was also being played out within the club.
We had the "totals",
the people with residual vision used to
take the piss out of the "totals".

The totals would experience camaraderie that would have issues with
the people with residual vision,
and the sports that took place were separated into
"totals" and "visuals".

It's like that in the black community sometimes…
When I was studying..
There is something called shadeism
you have communities that have issues with different shades of
black…
Is it?...
could it be that it is in our human nature too?
To find people who are the same us?

My conversations with Mike also reflect on how he felt whilst at a
school for the "blind" having some residual vision:

---

[1] People with some residual vision.

Mike: When I was at school,
a teacher came to the school, and
she was herself totally blind.

I was in the 6th form,
it was in the mid 80's.

This was the first time that I'd found somebody who'd really..
accepted me for who I was,
and we got on really well together.

It's a bit sad that we've lost touch,
but we did keep in touch for quite a long time,
and who knows when friendships re-emerge.

She was quite spiritual
I think had a quiet faith,
but a bit problematic with church (laughter).

There was the sense with her that
it was ok to be visually impaired.
She was musical as well,
so she encouraged me.

Sue: how did you know she accepted you when other people didn't?

I suppose that we shared something,
and she saw in me,
in some ways,
the "desperateness" of
feeling that I didn't fit in.

Sue: has this become less important now?

Certainly in relation to sight, yes.

I've just recalled something else;
and it sounds really awful..
but I remember occasionally getting to the stage
where..

My friend had other close visually impaired friends,
who I think; were either blind, or more or less blind,
and the bond they seemed to have
was something really special.

There were times that I wished that I would
wake up totally blind.

*Sue: so that you could belong to this group,
and have this bond.*

Yes. I think that there's a huge amount there about identity,
and that for me it has become easier because;
my identity at the end of the day,
is not about the impairments that I do or don't have,
but is about who I am in Christ.

Sue: so it's more about your spirituality now, rather than about having a visual impairment?

Yes. Yes.

I also receive emails from Patrick and Will about their experiences of living with blindness.

Email from Patrick:

Hi Sue,
I've been thinking a bit more about the whole question of being blind and what I said about vision not being something that I understood.

I think my pride in being "blind" is also about belonging, belonging to a community of people who live in the same way as I do. I don't have to explain to them about what it is like to go through life without sight, and what society's attitudes does to you when you are different. But the more I think about it the more I realise that as a group we never talk about feelings, or tolerate any negativity towards blindness, why is this I wonder? It's not that we are all men (I don't think men really do feelings very publicly whether they are sighted or blind!) there are women in our group too! I think partly it is our age and conditioning. Most of the people I stay in touch with went through the "blind school" process in the same way as I did, we were taught very firmly by sighted people about what the expectations would be for us as blind people, and in many ways that has made life easier. You have to be polite, make light of how blindness affects your life, and in doing this you are rewarded by not getting quite so much hassle!

I think I said to you before that sometimes I am not really sure that I want to share what my life is really like with the sighted world, it shakes everything up too much. Despite this ambivalence though I realise that dialogue is really important, and it is important for people such as myself to start being able to express how it really is rather than how the sighted world would like it to be for me.

Email from Will:

Hi Sue,
I wrote this quite recently and thought you might like to add it to your collection.

Blind,
yet having a certain amount of sight.
Fraud,
yet not having enough sight to get by with.
Terror
of losing the sight that I have and not being able to cope.
Longing
to belong to people who live the same kind of life
Hatred
of assumptions of what blind means to me.
Turmoil
stuck in the middle, without sight, without blindness.

Living in the Twilight Zone (Part Two)

If we define ourselves as either "blind" or "sighted" we find ourselves as Meredeth (2008) states "reduced" and marginalized, but by describing ourselves in a different way, could mean moving from a position of "either/or" to "both" which feels much more libratory. For me the term which resonates most is "partially sighted" in that it acknowledges both worlds and is more positive than "visually impaired" or having "low vision" which implies I am "less than" someone who is sighted, but I do not always experience this as a felt reality, it seems at times just a linguistic trick. As Kleege says, "Though I prefer the word *blind* I respect others who prefer *partially-sighted*. Perhaps it doesn't matter what words you use as long as you know what you mean" (Kleege 1999:41).

What seems to help me "feel" an identity which is both sighted and blind is when I hear the stories of other people who have similar, yet different experiences and these really resonate with my life experiences. For example, I have also noticed that the stories from my research which are now available in several mediums provoke intense responses from both blind and sighted people. As they listen (or read) the stories, they then tell their own stories, and this enriches both their own experience and that of ourselves.

Ray emailed me recently in response to reading Sarah's story in a recently published paper (Dale 2008a) and said:

"I think the worst thing about macular disease (which affects central vision) is that it takes away my sight and my dignity, but it doesn't give me any sense of belonging to the blind world. I can after all still see to walk into town, but having walked in to town, and gone into the shop I cannot see the products or the shop assistants' faces, or even what notes I have in my wallet. I just have to fight my way through the world being some kind of "non-being" with no culture that fits me, but reading Sarah's story I suddenly did not feel so alone any more, there were others out there, and perhaps they could be my new community".

Fitting in, feeling we are part of a group where other people have had similar life experiences normalises what we experience, and opens spaces for conversation across the divide of "sighted" and "blind". Because we stand across the divide, we can act as interpreters of both worlds, and help others re-define their lives. Also, as we hear other people's stories and they resonate with our own life experiences they enrich and able us to redefine how we describe our own lives.

PART 3

ENABLING PRACTICES
AND TRANSFORMING IDENTITIES

CHAPTER ELEVEN

EMOTIONAL SUPPORT

Within this chapter there is an exploration of what the emotional support needs may be for people who are visually impaired and it includes part one of the commentary entitled "developing emotional support services for people who are visually impaired"

What is meant by emotional support?

All of us need emotional support as we go through life, as John Donne commented "No man is an island entire of itself". Even if the emotional support is in the form of talking to a friend or going out with the lads, most of us from time to time need to talk with others about thoughts and feelings that are disturbing us. Whether we need more formal kinds of emotional support is dependent on: our existing relationships and support structures, our ability to access the above, and the severity of the turmoil we are experiencing. More formal emotional support can accessed in many different forms including telephone help lines, joining with others who are experiencing similar issues in a local support group, joining an on-line forum or accessing one of the talking therapies such as counselling or psychotherapy.

Most of us need more emotional support from others in situations where we face significant:

- Loss or bereavement – Losing something or someone that is precious to us can result in overwhelming feelings of sadness, despair and anger.

- Trauma – when we are subjected to situations that shock us or challenge everything we thought to be safe or true about life or our lives.

- Transition – Where we move from one life experience to another. To give a couple of examples; the life transitions we all experience from childhood to adolescence, from adolescence to adulthood, or transitions in our social or work experience; from working to unemployed, when our relationships with significant others encounters problems or changes.

- Oppression – where we feel that we have no control over our lives and others take no account of our needs and desires or we are socially excluded.

Needing emotional support from others from time to time in our lives does not, in my view, mean that we have mental health difficulties. If however we are unable to get the support that we need, at the time we encounter these difficulties, then this could lead to major problems such as acute anxiety or depression.

Research has shown us that people with a visual impairment are more likely to suffer from mental health issues such as depression than the general population (Burmedi et al. 2002; Nyman 2010b) but there is little research available to consider what it is about visual impairment that results in these mental health issues, and what we can do about it.

Losing sight or living with a visual impairment can lead a person to experiencing any or all of the above scenarios. Sight loss brings with it an experience of bereavement, as we have seen in the contributions of many within previous chapters. Loss of sight, loss of "who I was" (Sarah) loss of driving, loss of independence, loss of visual interaction with others. Many describe their diagnosis and treatment as "traumatic" and often display symptoms akin with post traumatic disorder "I keep having flashbacks of the moment he told me" (Stephen). "Every time I go for injections it gets worse, I feel deeply traumatised and afraid and have nightmares. It is like being tortured and told, 'It's for your own good' and yet nothing changes. I find myself often re-living the moment of the injections" (Annie). "I feel afraid all the time, sometimes I shake, it's like the world is a totally different place, one I don't know or like at all." (Peter).

People have often talked of "transition" feeling they are moving from a sighted world to a blind one. Some experience this in positive ways. George, for example, considers losing sight as a way for him to choose to engage with society in a different way "suddenly I had choices, I wasn't labelled as a junky or alcoholic, but as visually impaired. Strangely this gave lots of different possibilities". Others have found the transition extremely difficult. "I'm too old to start changing my ways, and actually I don't want to!" (Mo). Some (myself included) find themselves in between the worlds of the sighted and the blind. We do not have enough sight to get by in a sighted world, but we have too much to be considered truly blind. As Dennis's dilemma about using the white cane (chapter six) highlights "If I use the white cane, I feel a fraud because I'm not really blind, if I don't use it I am kidding myself that I am ok visually when I'm not". There are also changes and challenges in relationships for example when we move from the "carer" to the cared for.

Many people who are visually impaired, whether recently diagnosed or living with a visual impairment for a long time feel oppressed by their interactions with a society that has very negative attitudes towards visual impairment, they are often isolated and without a voice. As Tony comments in chapter two, many people feel marginalised, isolated and unable to change that position.

It would seem therefore a natural conclusion that visually impaired people would need some kind of emotional support (either informal or formal) at some time in their lives. I asked contributors what they thought about this and received a wave of responses:

Email from Michael:

Hi Sue,
I think what would have helped me was to have had some support when I was going through the treatment and diagnosis stage. Although the medical staff, were very professional, they did little beyond the physical care of my eyes. I would have liked to have had the opportunity to talk to someone about how I felt about this. I would like to have had time to process the information before I was discharged. I would have liked to have had information given to me about where I could find some support, e.g. contact details for a support group or even counselling service. I would have also liked my family to have more information about my condition and what this might mean for me psychologically as well as whether I was going to trip over the dog etc.

Email from Peter:

Dear Sue,
Thank you for your email –
As I think I said to you earlier, when you are diagnosed and registered it often feels like failure. I felt a failure. I had ceased to live up to having good eyesight and life expectations.

No-one ever asked me how I felt about all of this, it was just expected that I would engage with rehabilitation and get on with it. It meant that all my anger, sadness got buried and on the surface I did get on with it, but underneath I fell apart. Eventually I went to my GP who diagnosed depression, and gave me anti-depressants and offered counselling. The counsellor however did not get the sight loss issues at all. She thought they were totally separate from the depression.

I think that if I had been offered some kind of support alongside the medical treatment then I wouldn't have got so depressed. I just felt so alone with it all. It didn't even have to be formal counselling, just other people in similar situations who could listen, or share experiences. I also think that it would have been more helpful to have had a counsellor who understood about sight issues!

Conversations with Annie:

Sue: When you think back over this time..
What would have made it better do you think?

Annie: I think
to be honest...
the only thing that would have made it better was for someone to have told me that they could
make my sight better.
I couldn't think past that.
I just wanted my sight back.
When I was going to the hospital that was all I wanted.

The girl from social services didn't get it at all.
She thought giving me a white stick was brilliant.
I hated it!

I think afterwards it would have been helpful if my family had some counselling so they knew what to do with me.
They just made everything far worse,
didn't really understand what it was like for me at all.

Not only could I not see, but I felt really down,
I cried all the time,
I had nightmares where doctors continually held me down to perform operations on my eyes without anaesthetic.
I just felt nobody really understood what it was like for me.

I did have some telephone counselling with the RNIB some time later, and that was helpful,
mainly because the girl I spoke to was also
visually impaired.
If she hadn't been I think it would have been a waste of time.
I certainly wouldn't have gone to see a sighted counsellor.
I don't think I would have even talked to you,
because unless it happens to you..
it is too hard to understand.

Email from Emma:

Hi Sue,
Looking back I think that I probably did need someone to talk to about my feelings. It was hard growing up being classified by everyone as "not normal". School was ok because it was a school where everyone was visually impaired, but even there we had lots of

crap thrown at us by the sighted tutors about what blindness should or shouldn't mean. They did have a counselling service there but I didn't access it, again it was manned by sighted counsellors, and at that stage in life I thought all sighted people were idiots!

When I went through a very bad time at work I did access the work's counselling service, and actually she was really good, even though she wasn't visually impaired she didn't make assumptions, but I still would have preferred to have talked to someone that was visually impaired.

I think the problem is that unless you are visually impaired you don't really get it. It is outside your life experience.

Email from Will:

Hi Sue,
It is really interesting reading about the lack of counselling and psychological support for people in the UK. It doesn't really tie up with what happens here in New Zealand.

Within our local health board psychologists work alongside the ophthalmology staff such that people are assessed and offered whatever support is needed. I'm not sure they always take up the counselling services, but at least I suppose it is expected that they may need it.

I can't think how difficult it must be not to have psychological issues addressed at all as part of the eye health team! There has been criticism by many however that the linking of psychology with the ophthalmology department gives the impression that mental illness is linked with vision loss, and that as people often don't attend therapy sessions this should be lost.

I was offered therapy as a youngster, but declined! When I was older and trained as a therapist myself it was part of the course requirements, so I think it was only then I started to address my own issues.

Conversations with Pauline:

Pauline: the worst for me was just nobody listened
they didn't ever ask how I was coping,
I thought I was going mad,
the "Charles Bonnet" was not explained.
Anxiety was there all the time.
All the time.

If I managed to get to the supermarket….

Sue: it was really difficult?

Yes.
It wasn't that I just couldn't see the products,
it was that I used to get panic attacks,
feel as if I was going to die,
I thought that everyone was staring at me,
and would then be even more panic ridden
because I couldn't find the exit.

My family really did not understand – apart from wanting me to go in a home!

If I had been offered counselling I would have snapped it up.

I think my family also needed re-training so they knew a bit more about what I was going through.
All they saw was mum going mad.

Email from Caroline:

Hi Sue,
What emotional support would I have liked?

That's the one million dollar question I think. I suppose the stroppy part of me says that I shouldn't need any extra support just because I am visually impaired. I think what I really have always wanted and still want is for people just not to be so prejudiced and to treat me like a human being.

As that's not likely to happen I would like to be able to access someone to talk to from time to time who understands the visually impaired world, because at times living with a visual impairment is so frustrating. Preferably this would be someone who is also visually impaired!

I think that there also needs to be a change in the attitudes at eye clinics such that when families are delivered with the news that they are going to have to live with little or no vision they are supported – I know my family were totally traumatised by being told that their child would be blind, and I can imagine being told in later life would be no easier.

Developing Emotional Support Services for People who are Visually Impaired

As stated previously, all of us have times in our lives when we need emotional support, and this is often provided informally by friends and family. Isolation however is one of the most common issues cited by people who are visually impaired (Burmedi et al. 2002; Nyman, Gosney, and Victor 2010a). This sense of isolation could be due to mobility issues, age (the majority of people who are visually impaired are over 65 and have been affected also by other age related health problems (Hodge, Barr, and Knox 2010)) social factors; as we have seen in previous chapters societal attitudes often have a profound effect on how people who are visually impaired relate to sighted others. Many people who are visually impaired also live alone (Stephens 2007), both in the older age group where a partner may have died, but also in working age people where the proportion of single people is significantly higher than in their sighted peers. There are also issues regarding sighted friends and family members not being aware of the issues connected to living with low or no vision, or losing sight. This means that natural occasions for emotional support are often reduced. It seems imperative, therefore, to consider how professionals involved in services interacting with people who are visually impaired respond to this deficit.

This does not necessarily mean that everyone who is visually impaired "needs" counselling, or has a psychological problem, more that perhaps there should be more options available for people to access formal emotional support. If we consider losing sight as a transitional process (Thurston 2010) then different levels of emotional support will be needed at different stages of the visual impairment journey. (Thetford et al. 2008; Douglas, Pavey, and Corcoran 2008; Hodge, Barr, and Knox 2010). The RNIB is recently developing a "thresholds framework" clarifying levels of emotional support needed at different stages of the eye care pathway[1] which it is hoped will ensure that terminology is consistent across the field.

If diagnosis is the beginning of the sight loss journey then provision for emotional support should begin with ophthalmology clinics. Despite the recognition of this need (McBride 2005) and this being highlighted in various national standards and guidelines[2] it is rarely implemented effectively. Some changes have started to emerge, for example in some ophthalmology clinics ECLO[3] staff are appointed to support patients to provide "emotional support, advice and information, guidance about registration, explanation of eye conditions, family support and family support" (Seeing-Sense 2010). However most see their role as being involved with practical issues and few are trained in basic listening or counselling skills which would then enable them to support people emotionally. As Nyman comments, "the potential for ECLO's to provide emotional

---

[1] For more information see www.rnib.org.uk/emotional support service
[2] Low vision services consensus group 1999, NHS Eye Care Services Programme 2007, NICE 2004, Vision2020uk 2008
[3] Eye clinic liaison officers who currently provide information and liaise between clinicians and practical assistance within the ophthalmology department

support has yet to be realized. (Nyman, Gosney, and Victor 2010a:199).

Although there is some evidence of good practice in ophthalmology clinics with the majority of attendees being satisfied with the treatment they received (Douglas, Pavey, and Corcoran 2008) there are still people who find their consultants attitudes unhelpful (Vale 2001). One man (who would like to remain anonymous) told me "He (the consultant) would often come with his entourage of students and discuss me without even saying one word to me. I just felt as if they didn't see any purpose in talking to me at all, or listening to my concerns". Certainly this ties in with the experiences of several of the contributors to this book, and also my own. Surely the first step in emotional support is that we at least listen to people's concerns and acknowledge them as people rather than just conditions?

Although the focus of work within an eye clinic is on medical care and retaining sight, perhaps clinicians need to remain aware of the psychological impact that diagnosis and treatment has on their patients. One way of addressing this would be that when a diagnosis of untreatable sight loss is made it needs to be followed up by a psychosocial assessment which would identify both practical and emotional needs of the person such that appropriate referrals could be made. Improved training on the psychological impact of sight loss may also enable clinicians to support their patients better when delivering a life changing prognosis.

Thurston's (2010) participants identified a number of ways in which services for visual impairment including the need to close "the gap between diagnosis and social care, and placing the issue of disability more firmly on the political agenda" (Thurston 2010:8). Often people find themselves with a diagnosis and possibly registered as severely sight impaired (blind) or sight impaired (partially sighted) but once they are discharged by the hospital are not supported at all. Within some areas social services will follow up registration with a visit or information about services, but this does not happen routinely in all areas of the UK leaving many people unsure of any services in their area.

Despite the evidence that visual impairment has a "profound negative emotional impact on individuals" (Nyman, Gosney, and Victor 2010a; Burmedi et al. 2002) and that there is some evidence of a demand for emotional support that is not being met (Nyman, Gosney, and Victor 2010a) funding is often not available to set up sight specific services, this is partly because as yet there is no conclusive evidence of what kind of support enables people to have a better sense of emotional and social wellbeing (Nyman, Gosney, and Victor 2010a). Most of the services currently set up to support those who are visually impaired are run within the voluntary sector, and do not have the resources or expertise to run research projects as "random controlled trials" which are considered necessary to secure funding for treatment from NHS. To address some of these issues VINCE[4] (Visual Impairment Network of Counselling and Emotional Support) has been set up. This is a multi-agency network established to: Develop collaborative working between counsellors and emotional support service providers, share good practice, service developments, evaluation and research outcomes, influence the development of counselling and emotional support services for adults, children and families affected by sight loss.

In my view there needs to be a multi-tier approach to providing formal emotional support for those who are visually impaired provided over several years following diagnosis. This would include:

• Support being available within ophthalmology clinics at times of diagnosis, and registration. This could include better practices from clinicians, a psychosocial assessment to determine needs, improved ECLO provision, and signposting.

• Practical and emotional support being offered to both the person with the visual impairment and their family, together with opportunity for referral to sight specific support groups or counselling services.

• Funding for sight-loss specific therapeutic services, to include counselling, telephone support, peer support, therapeutic group and family support.

• Ongoing follow up and support for people and their families post-registration and discharge from hospital clinics to review needs.

---

[4] For more information about VINCE see www.vision2020uk.org listed under special interest groups

CHAPTER TWELVE

TALES FROM THE COUNSELLING ROOM

Following on from the previous chapter this chapter explores some of the contributor's experiences of using formal emotional support in the form of counselling, family and narrative therapy. It also includes part two of commentary entitled "developing emotional support services for people who are visually impaired".

Journal June 2008

I am coming to the end of my contract as senior counsellor and project co-ordinator for the RNIB counselling project in Bristol, and have just been completing the final report. The counselling statistics show that the service has been successful, both in terms of service user satisfaction, and in terms of showing clear evidence of clinical change[1].

I have learnt so much from my time working in this setting. It has challenged everything I thought I knew about visual impairment, and also everything I thought I knew about counselling.

I realised very soon into my work in Bristol that traditional counselling models I had learned did not really address many of the issues the people who were accessing the service were bringing. I needed to think outside the box so to speak. Whilst counselling gave people an opportunity to reflect on their inner world, what most of the people I had been meeting in Bristol had brought were issues related to their interaction with the outside world. Yes there were people who could and did use counselling to explore all the feelings surrounding sight loss and the trauma of diagnosis, but there were many others whose issues just did not fit into this kind of introspection. I looked more and more towards systemic, family and narrative therapies for ways of working that helped people re-negotiate their relationship with visual impairment and also with their friends and families and the sighted world.

There are estimated to be over 400 different models of counselling and therapy in the UK (Norcross 2005) and as we can see from the contributions in this book there are many different

---

[1] Dale (2008) Report on RNIB Bristol Counselling project 2005-2008.

experiences of losing sight and living with a visual impairment. There is also little evidence to show if any particular psychotherapeutic model is helpful (Nyman, Gosney, and Victor 2010a) so trying to identify one specific intervention that is appropriate for all visually impaired people would seem impossible. What has struck me forcibly, in my own personal practice as a counsellor working in this field, is that the psychotherapeutic models which consider people's sense of self and identity as something located deep within their genetic make up or history of life experiences and attachments does not always seem as helpful as approaches that see identity and self as socially constructed through relationship.

For the visually impaired person who is already experiencing "being trapped inside myself" (Andy) and who experiences the sighted world as oppressive; working in ways that solely focus on their inner world could mean that they are only able to find ways in which they can change this inner world in terms of thoughts, feelings and behaviours. It may not enable them to re-connect with the world around or challenge those sighted norms that are causing them to feel oppressed. It may also replicate the experience of visual impairment which often isolates the person from community in which they live and work.

Losing sight often seems to mean loss of contact with the external world. Adam comments of his experience of degenerating sight:

> Adam: The whole journey all my life
> 　　as regards my sight loss
> has **absolutely**
> put me inside.
>
> The relationship I have with my internal world is ...
> increasing,
> and is already very, very, very strong.
> It is increasing,

Sarah comments on her experience of counselling:

> Sarah: I think because sight loss was so new to me
> and I was experiencing so much loss,
> I had to work through these feelings of
> despair and anger,
> get in touch with my "inner me"
> before I could start to negotiate my relationships with others.
> Working with you
> in a counselling setting focussed me in doing this.
> What happened then though was I suddenly realised

that this was all very well,
but other people were a real problem,
treating me so differently from before
and the isolation of that..
not knowing what to do about that felt like
I was trapped,
and however well I knew the "inner me"
this wouldn't change.

I think what helped with that
were the research conversations we then had.
Telling my story to others.
This put me in touch with Andy and others,
this helped me find a new place for myself in the world.
I described it I think when we talked as like "knitting in the dark",
which was a bit chaotic and scary,
but the new garment that emerged was worth it.

Comments from client evaluation forms (completed at the end of counselling) within the RNIB Bristol Counselling project 2005-2008 reported few negatives – apart from the desire for more sessions:

"Counselling helped me to deal with the issues my sight loss raised within my family and especially its impact on my son"

"Counselling has helped me deal with the frustration that I felt towards my family when they fuss over me after my sight loss. Counselling helped me to work out a different way of dealing with the situation so that conflict could be avoided"

"Helped me to deal/come to terms with issues around parent's death" (Dale 2008).

Claire wrote to me in response to listening to "knitting in the dark" (Dale 2006) whilst on an information day at the RNIB. She had recently worked with a counsellor from one of the sight-loss specific telephone services:

Dear Susan Dale,
Having listened to your "knitting in the dark" stories while I was on a course at the local blind society I asked for your contact details, because I wanted to write to tell you how helpful they were. I realised that my own feelings were not so crazy after all.

I have just finished working with a counsellor on the telephone, and having her listen to me was very important to me. I think I felt totally overwhelmed by losing sight and couldn't see any ways forward. I just felt so depressed and down, and even at times that life wasn't worth anything. Counselling really helped me and gave me the space to say how I felt. It has helped me a lot to come to terms with what was a terrible loss. My only criticism was that it ended too soon. I would have liked more sessions but realised that there were so many other people wanting support this wouldn't be fair.

I have thought about seeing a counsellor privately, but I guess I am just a bit scared that they wouldn't understand.

I wanted to write to you because I understand you are involved with trying to set up more services for people like me, and my telephone counsellor thought you might be interested in what I had to say.

The more stories I heard during the course of my work, the more I recognised the need for people with a visual impairment both to have people available to listen empathically (especially at the time of diagnosis) and also ways of re-negotiating their relationships with those around them. I wanted to find a way of helping people relate better to their partners, families and friends such that there was a better understanding of what living with a visual impairment may mean. I turned for inspiration to the systemic and family therapy fields.

Family and group therapists have recognised this need to re-negotiate relationships and developed therapeutic models that centre the "relationship" in the process rather than the individual, and then work with the couple or group to find new ways of relating. This seemed to be very appropriate for some of the families who wanted to understand their relationships where one of them had lost sight, and also ties in with some research where participants have identified the need for family support (Douglas, Pavey, and Corcoran 2008; Thurston 2010; Nyman, Gosney, and Victor 2010a).

Email from Beth:

Hi Sue,
Thank you for your email, I am really excited about your forthcoming book. You asked me whether there was anything that helped when I was first diagnosed with glaucoma and macular disease.

Initially I had some telephone counselling from the RNIB, this helped me in that they told about Charles Bonnet syndrome and in the early days helped with the panic. When that finished I went with my husband and son to see a Relate[2] counsellor for family therapy. There was just so much going on for me that my husband and son didn't seem to understand at all and I was scared we would end up divorced. I thought we could talk about it with a referee so to speak. This was probably the best thing that we as a family have ever done. I realised through this that although this was an awful thing for me,

---

[2] Relate is a counselling organisation specifically offering couples and family therapy.

it was probably just as awful for my family for they had lost the mum/wife who used to hold the family together, I was a completely different person. We had six sessions altogether and all of us were able to have our say and say how this thing had affected us. If anything I think we are now closer than we were before. My son who is now 19 and now at university says that he accessed the college counsellor when things were getting on top of him which he would never have done without the good experience he had at Relate.

Working with couples and families began to become integral to my work, but there still seemed something missing. Group work also seemed appropriate as it engaged people with each other and the outside world. Annie comments of her experience of attending a "finding your feet"[3] weekend run by the RNIB:

> Annie: Going to this hotel that was designed for people like me with little vision with my daughter was great.
> Talking to other people who had the same problems,
> sharing my worst fears,
> it helped my daughter as well
> understand a bit more about what it was like for me.
> It kind of felt like I had found a new group of friends
> I felt less mad..
> if that makes any sense.

Michael emails me about his attendance of a peer support group run by his local society.

> Hi Sue,
> You asked what helped me most after I had been diagnosed, well I think that it was probably the "blind club" run by the local society here. It would have been good if it was a bit more structured and someone had been there to help us talk about the things that were getting us down, but it did give us an opportunity to be with others who faced the same challenges and have a natter and a cup of tea.

Even informal groups not specifically set up as "therapy" were having a very therapeutic effect, and this seemed to address issues of isolation and enable people with similar life experiences to talk together. I was also aware however of a need to find an intervention that enabled what seemed to be sometimes silenced and isolated individuals to develop a voice that was listened to.

I learnt about narrative therapy whilst undertaking my Master's degree in counselling at Bristol University. Narrative therapy comes from a position of seeing reality as socially constructed within

---

[3] For more information about the RNIB "finding your feet" see http://www.rnib.org.uk/livingwithsightloss/Documents/FYF_striding_about _prog.doc.

relationship and the stories we tell about our lives. Its aims are very simple; to enable people to move from telling thin problem saturated stories to thick rich descriptions of their lives (White and Epston 1990). The role of the counsellor (or therapist) is not that of an expert, but decentred.

Narrative therapy grew out of the work of family therapists working in Australia, and moved beyond holding the relationship of specific individuals within a therapeutic setting.[4] This started to enable people from fragmented communities to re-author their lives by linking with others across common themes in a process called outsider witness practices or definitional ceremony[5]. Narrative therapists also located the "problem" that people brought to the therapeutic encounter outside the person and used what they described as "externalising conversations" (White 1985). This enabled people to stand outside the problem to consider the effect it was having on their lives.

What follows first is an excerpt from my work with a couple (May and Peter) that uses externalising conversations to explore their relationship with blindness.

The Grilling of Mr B[6]

May and her husband had requested to meet with me following May's diagnosis of Age related macular degeneration (AMD) which had resulted in May losing most of her central vision and her being registered as seriously sight impaired (blind). They both considered that "blindness" was affecting May's confidence, making her depressed and was "coming between them". May was unsure about counselling thinking that "all that touchy feely stuff isn't really for me. We were always told 'stiff upper lip' and got on with it".

Some weeks later when May had spoken again about how "blindness" was really getting her down, and "upsetting Peter". 'It's like this malevolent person has come into our lives'. I told them how interested I was in the tactics used by this malevolent person to disrupt their lives and asked whether we could interview him (or her) in some way.

There was a significant pause (I thought O my God have I got

---

[4] For more information about narrative therapy see the works of White and Epston (1990).
[5] There are fuller descriptions of these practices both in the introduction and also within chapter fourteen.
[6] The Grilling of Mr B was first published as a journal article in "Therapy Today" September 2009 (20)7 and is included here with permission.

this right) and then there was laughter.

They both became animated entering into the playfulness of the suggestion "grilling Mr B" said May "I would really love to give him a good grilling". We looked at possibilities as to how this might work and made plans for the following week.

May decided that she would like "the black chair" to be occupied by Peter who would act the part of Mr B (because he is a brilliant actor), and that it would be me who interviewed him (she would whisper to me with suggestions if I didn't know what to ask).

She thought that she would then like to be interviewed by me as to whether she recognised the "tactics" which Mr B employed and the kinds of "weapons" she had to "fight with him". What follows is a small excerpt of the script which I recorded (audio) for May and Peter to have a record of the occasion. Our conversation was not as neat as it appears below; there were a lot of pauses, laugher, stutters and umms... and ehrs... which I have removed to make the transcript more accessible to readers, and of course this is just a snippet of a much longer conversation. The transcript is not the entirety of the event, only a shadow of something that has gone and indeed within the telling it becomes something new.

The Grilling of Mr B (the interview)

S: Mr B you are charged with disrupting the lives of May and Peter. Is this true?

Mr B: Yes. Oh Yes. I have been quite successful (looks smug)

S: They are a couple who have lived together for nearly fifty years, and survived so many ups and downs in their lives, a world war, raising of children, losing their son, cancer, but I am informed that none of these were so disruptive as you have been.

How have you managed to achieve this disruption when so many others have failed?

Mr B: I eat away at May's self confidence. It's not really that hard.

S: You eat away at her self confidence? How do you do that?

Mr B: I tell her she is useless. It's easy really.

S: You tell her she is useless. May is a very
resourceful woman, why I wonder do you think she believes you?

Mr B: I am very convincing. I cash in on the fact that part of her body is not working, the part she values most. Her eyes. I keep her shut into a world others can't share. I stop her seeing the expressions on other people's faces. I trap her into a world where there is just me and her.
So she listens, because….. I'm all she's got.

S: So you trap her in a place where she is separated from Peter and others that care for her.

Mr B: Yes. When she is alone ..she listens best then.

S: Is there anyone/anything else who helps you with this "trapping".

Mr B: Yes. I have hundreds of people everywhere that help.

S: That sounds like a big boast.

Mr. B: It's true. Most people are scared of being blind. They fear blindness more than anything. It is their worst fear, going blind, getting old so they pity, patronize and avoid people who carry my calling card.

S: Your calling card?

Mr B: The white cane of course

S: Oh… (I feel totally lost for words)
Is there anyone else?

Mr B: The professionals at the eye hospital help too. They tell people "there is nothing we can do. You are untreatable". Their expertise and inability to "do anything" and their acceptance of failure convinces May that she is powerless.

S: You seem to think you are invincible. Surely that isn't true?

Mr B: I succeed because I keep people isolated and afraid, they cannot see beyond that. Of course I am invincible……

This is only a brief excerpt of the grilling of Mr B. When May thought she had answers to all the questions she wanted asked, I asked her about what she had heard to find out whether there were any clues to the "demolishment" (May's word) of Mr. B's power.

She reported being surprised at how accurate Mr. B's account was of the effects he had on her life, and that firstly she'd been angry with him, then amused (he seemed a very laughable figure) then sad and determined. Sad because of the way she had allowed him to isolate her from people who could support her like Peter and her many friends. Determined in that she could now see ways of avoiding his influence.

She also felt that Mr B wasn't actually "the blindness". Blindness was "different...a physical thing which I can learn to live with" Mr B was in fact "unmasked as fear" and that fear was not about the blindness itself but about "other peoples attitudes. How I felt about myself. Confidence that I could learn new skills at such an old age" and also "about dying – is this the beginning of the end?".

I asked May how she felt about the grilling of Mr. B "Amazed, now I can see him for what he is and I've stopped feeling that fluttery fear feeling inside. He is well and truly grilled ...and eaten".

We talked further about Peter and May's experience and what it was like for Peter to act the part of Mr. B. May said "It was a fun way of approaching something really serious. I'm not very good at all this 'how do you feel about it?' stuff. I suppose I come from an era of saying 'don't waste time crying' – and just get on with it". "I am amazed at how much we really knew about all of this" said Peter.

Within the externalising conversation "the grilling of Mr. B" May was able to systematically examine the effects that "blindness" had had on her life and even separate "blindness" from "Mr B" and how she could resist and redefine how she related with this "bloody problem". Both Peter and May had commented that "blindness had come between them, and was causing a 'rift' in their relationship", and that following this particular conversation they had become "closer and working together again". They both felt that because the conversation was "light and fun" it helped them move from being "entrenched in doom and gloom and only seeing the problem" to engaging with a therapeutic process in ways they had not thought possible. As White and Epston comment: externalising conversations "free persons to take a lighter, more effective less stressed approach to 'deadly serious' problems, and present options for dialogue rather than monologue about the problem" (White and Epston 1990:40).

As I wrote this story I was aware that the writing did not constitute the reality of what happened between myself, Peter and May, but was only a reflection of how it was remembered now, and that may change! But it is hoped that the "grilling" enabled one person to research the influence of blindness in her life and to open up choices as to who she wanted to become in relation to this blindness. To a wider audience it enables a unique glimpse into the lived experience of a couple (both in their 80's) who had been affected by blindness, showing how medical understandings of sight loss and blindness "imprisoned" (May's description) May into a fixed identity, whereas blindness is in fact only part of who she is as a person.

Following the publication of, "the grilling of Mr. B" I received many emails, including several from people who were visually impaired some of whom had accessed the article via their counsellors and other contributors who regularly read work written by me.

Email from Will:

Hi Sue,
Just loved the article!
I have never really been sure that counselling works (or is wanted) by visually impaired people – how wrong was I!

I think what really resonated for me was that this kind of approach did not need May to "hang all her dirty washing out" so to speak. It sounds as if she really didn't want to talk at all about her feelings or all the things that had happened to her in the past. She just wanted not to be troubled by this Mr. B! and this is what she got.

Email from Patrick:

Hi Sue,
I have never believed that counselling would be the right option for me, but reading your article about Mr. B I wished that someone could have had that kind of conversation with me, many years ago.

I have always thought that a sighted counsellor would try to make me believe that I was somehow responsible for the feelings of rage I sometimes have towards a society that treats me so patronisingly. Perhaps she or he would have been right to do so; after all most sighted people actually do not realise they are acting patronisingly so what right have I to rage against them?

Email from Maria:

Hi Sue,
As I think I said to you before, I did not have a very good experience of counselling. I think this is partly due to the counsellor not having any idea what it was like to live with a disability, and the unfairness that you face every day of your life. I think it was also partly due to my expectation that she would be able to enable me to stop the

prejudice, which of course she couldn't. When I read your article about Mr. B I really wished that I had a counsellor who took this kind of approach. It didn't require (as my counsellor did) you to rake over all of the past and your childhood etc. etc. it just seemed to help both her and her husband think about her disability in a different way, and that was all that was needed.

Perhaps it would be helpful if counselling services were set up specifically for people with disabilities (especially vision problems) in mind?

Developing Emotional Support Services for People who are Visually Impaired (Part Two)

As stated in the previous chapter I consider that formal emotional support services for people who are visually impaired should be multi-tiered with the first considerations taking place within eye clinics especially at the times of diagnosis and registration, then there should be a range of support strategies available for people as they make the transition from sighted to living as someone who is visually impaired. Currently these services are very fragmented due both to little evidence of what kind of service needs to be in place, and lack of central funding. The project I was involved with in Bristol was funded by the Department of Health, but only for three years as a pilot project, following this funding was dependent on the charity which hosted it, and fundraising, and survival of this and that of other such projects is tenuous.

Thinking of what model of support would be appropriate for visual impairment I have turned to services set up to support other specific groups to see what works. Some of the most relevant fields seem to be those which are set up to support people who have been affected by other health related issues. I have also been very interested in reading research undertaken in Wales (where I live) relating to substance abuse and how people can be supported. The emphasis here is put on "psychosocial interventions". Within the substance abuse field there is clear evidence that the combination of practical social interventions combined with psychotherapeutic support were much more effective than either intervention on its own (Davies 2007). The author comments that this combined approach,

"is not exclusive to substance misuse issues but can also be provided in the context of other health, social and life issues faced by people"(Davies 2007:1).

Indeed we see within other health related issues such as coronary care and oncology departments care provided that includes both practical and emotional support. Should this kind of intervention be available for those affected by sight loss? After all people losing sight need rehabilitation and information as well as emotional support. Guide Dogs have recently piloted a scheme they have called "The Middle Step" (Freeman 2009) which clearly showed that the inclusion of emotional support improved the functionality and wellbeing of visually impaired people and clearly accentuated the need for psychosocial interventions.

If we can provide the robust research, and evidence of the kind that the substance abuse psychologists cited, then we may be in a better position to acquire the necessary funding to provide psychosocial interventions to people who are visually impaired. Unfortunately whereas substance misuse has strong government backing the needs of visually impaired people are, it seems, of less political interest both to governments and the general public.

Currently counselling, support groups and family therapy for people who are visually impaired are provided almost exclusively by the voluntary sector, and funding for such projects is continually difficult, especially in times of recession and where a lot of funding (such as the Lottery) is being shifted to cover specific projects (currently the 2012 Olympics) and the remainder spread thinly to cover lost statutory funding in many strategic areas of social support. Unless national or local government commissions, or takes a strategic decision, to actively support the emotional and psychological needs of visually impaired people the voluntary sector will need to continue to provide these services and therefore the support received will depend on where you live and how active the local society or branch of national charity is. Currently in the rural part of Wales in which I live there is no support for visually impaired people beyond rehabilitation services, and then there is sometimes a three year wait.

There is a need for co-ordinated research efforts to enable an evidence base to be constructed that gives evidence of what people with a visual impairment experience, and what they would consider helpful in terms of emotional support. There is also a need to collate data showing what kind of intervention or range of interventions is effective and longitudinal studies showing whether these have any impact on mental health and wellbeing in this group of people. There could also be more extensive reviews of psychosocial support found effective with other health related groups such as oncology, coronary care and substance misuse which could be used to link to the needs of people who are visually impaired.

Specifically regarding counselling services for people who are visually impaired, the pilot projects set up to assess therapeutic value have all shown that people have both appreciated the service given, and there is evidence of a reduction in psychological distress (Hodge, Barr, and Knox 2010; Dale 2008; Nicholls 2004). None of these studies however addressed the model of counselling provided although apart from my own work most of the counsellors adopted a "humanistic" stance[7] in their therapeutic work. As stated above, although I value this approach, I am conscious of its limitations when working with clients who bring issues relating to negative attitudes of the society in which they live.

Beth sends me a poem:

"How do you feel" said the counsellor?
How would you feel if crap was thrown at you all the time?
But how do you feel?
How would you feel if the crap kept coming
and there is nothing you can do about it?
But how do you feel?
How would you feel if someone could say the crap throwing isn't fair
but did nothing to protect you?
But how do you feel?
Angry, upset and ….
I'm off!!

McLeod and Cooper speak of the need for a pluralistic approach to counselling and psychotherapy (McLeod and Cooper 2010) with emphasis on diversity of approaches being available for diverse needs and I am sure that this kind of thinking will be beneficial, especially within a field such as that of visual impairment where people have such diverse needs at different stages of their journey into visual impairment.

The other issue highlighted by contributors and also cited within Thurston's (2010) study is the comment from visually impaired people that sighted counsellors may not be of any help. As Caroline wonders "would a sighted counsellor have any understanding of my world? You can only understand it if you live it I think."

I am certainly not advocating that only counsellors who are visually impaired should work with people who are visually impaired, but I think perhaps we need to look behind the comment to understand better why people might think in this way, certainly it is not unusual for people to want to work with a counsellor who has faced or face similar issues to their own. For example many substance misuse workers are people who have experienced

---

[7] the humanistic approach can be described as emphasising the capacity of an individual for personal growth and development.

addiction issues, or often female clients will request a female counsellor. What perhaps we need to identify is how meaningful dialogue can take place between people who are sighted and visually impaired about their needs; such that there is less misunderstanding and prejudice. After all, just as not all people with a visual impairment fit into the stereo type image of "blind", neither are all people who are sighted prejudiced about what it could mean to live with a visual impairment.

CHAPTER THIRTEEN

JOINED UP VOICES

This chapter uses excerpts from group conversations between people who are visually impaired to explore what moves them from feeling isolated, marginalised and without a voice to a vibrant community who have a degree of control over services and how they interact with sighted communities.

Journal 21st January 2008

We did it! What an amazing experience.
In all my years as a therapist I don't think that I have ever experienced a group process in quite the same way. Just making it to the location by way of foot, train, bus was a major challenge. Even finding the room was difficult, and as for discovering the gents… fortunately not my remit!

And our conversations ….well – they just took my breath away!

The relationship I have with these four men is something I have not experienced before. I assumed that it would be like the "counselling" relationship which is intense, but you always know that it will end, and it is held separate from the rest of your life.

This is different. The intensity is there. Our lives feel woven together, but, it crosses the boundaries. These people are part of my life now. We have become friends, and although that is quite wonderful, it is not what I expected and has made me aware that undertaking this kind of research is not something to be taken on lightly or with the thought that it will end with the submission of the paper. It has transformed the whole of my life, not just the academic!

The meeting I describe in my journal above was between myself and four men; Mike, Dennis, Adam and Tony who were involved in my doctoral research project. Some may wonder at the inclusion of what on the surface seems an ordinary meeting, but, meetings between those of us who are visually impaired are rare. We are a minority group and rarely have the opportunity to be together, and talk specifically, about things appertaining to visual impairment.

Normally meetings of this kind do not happen without the intervention of sighted people. It was an extraordinary morning! What follows are excerpts from our group conversation which are presented in the form of a drama:

Conversations between Sue, Adam, Dennis, Mike and Tony
Act I

Stage directions:

Four men and one woman are seated in the corner of a large rather shabby university room. They have been sitting there for about two hours engaged in heated discussion about their experiences of living with a visual impairment and the relationship they have with sighted others. A collection of white canes are propped against the wall along with coats and a collection of half empty coffee cups.

The woman looks rather nervous. She has been trying to read from her laptop computer emails sent to her in response to the stories they have been compiling of their lives. There has been much laughter both at her inaptitude at reading aloud, and also regarding the contributions. Now however the room is ominously silent..

Sue: So, what's your feelings?
I was really scared,
I mean I've loved working with all of you
and have written...
but sending our stories out to other people,
even though they're people I know well.

There's this kind of terror sending these out
into the void
and waiting.
Are people going to be really critical?
are they going to be...?
but actually I think what people told were positive and kind of affirmed...
What's it like for you?

Dennis: It's really nice to hear independent feedback.
It's quite affirming to hear individuals say,
"I can relate to that".
Because I think one of the issues that comes up for many people with
a sight problem..
Is isolation.
It gradually starts to take that away.

And it's really good to hear the number of people who really did echo what all of us said.

I found that quite, even..
almost uplifting
to hear that was really good.

Mike: There are a couple of things..
The last email[1]...
I actually find quite offensive.
It was written to you, so as a friend she or he feels
he can say these things..
Because it says,
stories don't matter,
and it's not real research
and..
I just think
as Adam says it probably says more about her than us
but...

Sue: But it still hurts in a way.
And it hurts when I send articles and they say:
"it's not real counselling"
or not "real research"
That still hurts.

Tony: Because they've got a narrow view of what research is..

Sue: Yes. They've got a narrow view
and I do try to take the view that it says something about
them rather than me!

Mike: And people are so often looking for quantitative research and
thinking about numbers,
you know..
One hundred people say this and a thousand say that
and that's what matters.
That's what RNIB would say

(Lots of group affirmations and laughter)

Dennis: I'm glazing over already!

Tony: They think the researcher should be wearing a long white coat,
or glasses halfway down...

(Group laughter)

Mike: The other thing that struck me was Pat's response..

---

[1] This was an email from a sighted friend who had told me in no uncertain terms that I ought to give up on narrative research as the stories were too "gut wrenching" and that I ought to undertake a "proper research project".

Sue: The ophthalmologist? Shall I re-read the email?

Mike: Yes.

Sue:
Email from Pat

Hi Sue,
When I was a ten, my mother started to have problems with her eyes. I remember her going backwards and forwards from the hospital, and her being very sad and feeling scared.

"They can't do anything for my eyes" she said to me. "You will just have to get on with life on your own now". She kind of faded away after that, just gave up on life I suppose, in hindsight I guess she was depressed. But I didn't really understand then, but I do remember deciding that I would one day become a great eye surgeon and make sure no-one else lost their sight and suffered like this.

I have now been an ophthalmologist for many years, and I have more realistic goals, but I hope that I have always tried to treat people as more than just "a pair of eyes" but I guess that I have never really thought about vision in anything other than medical terms. These narratives are not really about vision at all, and they trouble me, make me feel I am missing something. Perhaps I feel excluded and don't really get it, and perhaps I feel you haven't even tried to think about this from my perspective. How could I possibly do more? What do you want of me?

Yet despite the anger which I guess is a bit defensive, I want you all to keep writing, and I want to understand.

I stood looking at all the people sitting waiting in the clinic the other day, and thought about what their life experiences might be and I was afraid. Very afraid, yet hopeful.

That's the end of the email...

Mike: I heard quoted a priest,
an Anglican priest
who was getting very fed up of working for the church and she came up with the phrase which says,
"I want out of the belief business and into the behold business".
And if I translate it to this context:
"I want out of the understanding business
and into the beholding business".

i.e. I don't want people to understand and **do things,**
I want people to behold my experiences
and the experiences of others,
and to respect them.

Sue: we can never fully understand can we…..?

Mike: and not have to think they understand them.
But so often..
and that's sometimes the trouble with training packages,
that are put together to try and help people
understand sight loss
I just want people to …
behold it.
Respect it.

Dennis: How do we get there?..

Mike: I think it's the whole training method that needs to change.
Organisations like to put together packages that we can deliver
in a lunch hour or whatever..
and so much of life in our culture is about
eliminating mystery
and I think in this work as well
we're saying there is a mystery about visual impairment
because we are all unique
and we respond to it in different ways
and we need to somehow put that back in.
Because unless people are willing to accept that there's a mystery
around it because there are so many different variables..
We're going to prolong prejudices.

Sue: However hard I try,
and I've worked as a counsellor for many years
I can never ever say that I fully understand
the person that I am talking with.
Even if I think of people I have worked with for
years and years.
Because you cannot be them.

I rather like that idea that you can behold and respect
and hold their experience as being precious.

Tony: You can probably get partially inside the experience
but not 100% because it is not your experience, is it?
We've all got different experiences.

Sue: That email from Pat particularly struck me
because I thought,
"she's worked all these years and never actually thought..
how they might live their lives outside that consulting time".

I think she is quite angry actually…
Quite angry with me for disturbing her peace.

Where there any other stories which resonated? I could hear you
laughing…

Tony: Not laughing in derision
but certain resonance.
A humorous resonance.
You've got to see the funny side of it sometimes
Even though it might be difficult.

Training Packages...
any form of packaging is...
It's not about food is it?
It is not a package of cereal?
Why has everything got to be done up as a
certain kind of package?

Adam: We come from an education system
which teaches and doesn't allow people to learn!

Most of the emails felt quite validating..
and hearing my name mentioned by Will
I can just totally connect with that feeling of
sheer, excitement,
when you think or feel somebody has had
a similar experience.
But some of the comments from the sighted people....
like Mike said...

Mike: What made you feel the need to send the stories to sighted
people as well as visually impaired people Sue?

Sue: I suppose I thought I shouldn't be so ....
I was going to say "racist"...prejudiced.

I have conversations with people who are sighted
who have been very supportive
and I valued their kind of "take" on it
from a sighted perspective.
Because there was a criticism of my writing once..
This particular person, she thought I was ganging up against sighted
people.

Perhaps it was a mistake..
I don't know.

Mike: I'm not saying it was a mistake,
and I was just wondering what the process was
because there is a very different response.
The people who were visually impaired who responded,
they may not kind of agree with any of the stuff I said,
or any of the others said,
but it feels different.

Sue: Yes. The responses are different aren't they?
I mean the people who are visually impaired

there is a common connection
whereas, the people that have responded who are sighted
have actually made a judgement call on it.
I'm evaluating this about you.
But it hasn't elicited the personal stories.

Mike: Does that go then beyond the narrative
once you start drawing in people from beyond the narrative?

Sue: I don't know.
I suppose it depends whether you think the narratives
are about blindness
or about sight.

What I think I have learned
how far I've got
is that I am sighted and I am blind.
I think I can stand on either side of the fence of that one.
But I think more and more I am coming on the blind side,
because actually that feels a more comfortable place to be.

Tony: I think that we're all on both sides of the fence to a certain
degree.

Sue: I think what I've also learned about myself is that pragmatically
it is easier for me to make light of my visual impairment,
if I don't worry the sighted community with my difference.

I think....
going back to your original question
"why did I send our writing to sighted people"
I know that sighted people are going to read it
and I wanted I suppose to gauge what the impact might be,
what criticism I might get.

Dennis: You can't
You won't get the kind of criticism you get from them
from other visually impaired people.

Sue: Usually the visually impaired community
they might not agree with what I say
which is fine
but they are usually really supportive of people being empowered...
Whereas I am not sure that is always the case with the
sighted community.

Dennis: I think that it comes back to,
for want of a better expression,
we're in the same club.
Whereas once we talk about sighted people,
it's the masses.
By far.

Yet the one thing we've all got in common
that they don't have is the visual impairment itself.
So they will never be in our club.
But we want to be in theirs, kind of thing, because what we ultimately want
and the word that entered my head
when we talked about two letters from sighted people was integration.
Is that not what we ultimately want?

Just to be accepted as another Jo public who happens to have a sight problem?

Tony: I couldn't agree more!
I think this problem of..
putting people into brackets,
or boxes,
is not always very helpful is it?
I want to get on with people as people.

Dennis: I used to belong to a group
of visually impaired counsellors
and there was one particular lady there
and she absolutely hated hearing the expression "the blind".
Whenever it was in the press or the media,
or even in society generally.
She hated "the blind".

(Group laughter)

Sue: I can't say I'm very enamoured with it either!

Mike: I think the point you're saying as well Tony,
that we are people with a visual impairment,
not visually impaired people.
It makes a big difference!

When you said about integration
I was sitting here thinking
Yes.
Great idea!

Something we should all go for,
but...
Should we?

Because on one level.
Yes.
But actually in a sense
what we are experiencing today...
we are all experiencing something that
we might describe as special,

in a kind of non-patronising sense of the word
because we are in the same club...

Dennis: And I think that might be exactly where we are
at the moment,
today,
in England.

Mike: I suppose I am saying that to me
this does not feel a bad place to be.
I think for me,
integrating
yes, it is important
but also being able to stand by my identity
as someone with a visual impairment
as a gay man
as a person trying to discover faith
whatever it is..

Dennis: and all you really want is for others
to respect that.
But, nevertheless,
we're still going to leave this room today,
go out there into the world where sighted people are,
want to use the same services as them
want to get on with life the same as them.

Mike: Absolutely,

Dennis: Ultimately...
Perhaps integration is a bit idealistic at the moment!

I grew up in the 1950's in the back streets of south London
where if you were either,
gay, black, or as it was then, Irish,
you were absolutely laughed at.
You were driven out of the community
you were persona non grata..

(Group yes..yes..yes)

Dennis: and disabled,
disabled people were ridiculed
I think earlier Tony you used the word "spas"
which was common..
And I grew up in that community as a non-disabled person
when I think back on that
I feel quite uncomfortable.

Tony: To be quite honest.
as you said,

the word "spas" and other similar types of words was in common parlance
even for people who did not have that condition.
It could be someone with a learning disability,
or on the slow side..

Dennis: Visual Impairment wasn't an expression that existed.
It was blind!
Blind people were pitied.
They were pitied
"Oh they belong in a home" and that was that.

Adam: I think like so many things in life
there's a paradox
and I think that
although some of the things that we are talking about today
are not exclusive to our club,
or our 'ism, or our minority group, or whatever....
I do also think that there's a lot
that is specific to certain cultures.
There are some things that are specific to sight loss
as there are with the deaf community,
and finding that paradoxical balance
and understanding is something which I think demands
a greater sense of sensitivity.....

Something I am curious to know Sue
Or hear your process more is,
you've been quite safe in as much that you kind of
sit on the fence regarding sight and visual impairment.
You've got your awareness in both camps,
but inevitably there must have been times where one camp has been hooked more than the other
as a result of a particular experience?

Sue: I think working for the RNIB took me off the fence!

(Group laughter)

Sue: because up 'til then I had just gone along with the fact that I wasn't sighted
but I kind of acted as if I was sighted all the time,
and I think that more and more I am not prepared to do that
even if it makes it difficult for me
which it does often.

I am not prepared to do it any more
so my friends and family are having quite a rough time
at the moment
because I won't go along with things
that I would have done in the past.
So I think for me it has been therapeutic.

Dennis: But I think you have started something and
I'm not sure where it will finish.
When your dissertation is submitted,
and the process at the university finishes..
You have talked about presenting this...
That's where it goes to a different level!

Mike: The key thing I feel really passionate about,
is just the very fact that I feel..
it's true of disabled people generally,
but I think it is especially true of blind and partially sighted people that
we very rarely have an opportunity to have a voice.
And if we do have a voice,
it's often
given
by somebody else
it's not something that we seem able to be able to do ourselves because,
working with visually impaired people
is a multimillion pound business
and it sickens me
to be honest.

Sue: Do you think that there's something about the way we work
with something about us as blind and partially sighted people ..
That we don't fight for a voice?

In the same way..
I know that the deaf community very much fights for a voice?

Mike: And I think there's a very basic
practical reason for that
is that for deaf people
deaf people gather because they see each other
and you spot each another
and your means of communication is visual
so it draws people together.
If you're blind or partially sighted
often you need the mediation of someone else
to know that somebody is there
by which time that's happened
the opportunity's gone.

Just because I am blind or partially sighted
doesn't make me a good theologian,
it does not make me a good communicator,
it does not make me a good researcher,
but we've got to start somewhere
and that I think is what I feel passionate about..

What's come out of this study so far

is the amount of skill,
the amount of passion,
the amount of academic knowledge,
whether that be formal or informal
that comes out of it
and just shows that given the right environment
and the right tools
what we can do   for ourselves.

Following these conversations the dissertation was indeed submitted, primarily in audio format, which was intended to challenge the predominance of text within academic practices. Presenting the emerging narrative at conferences, and indeed incorporating these stories and others within a book has indeed taken the research to a new level. I also made the decision that although I had responses to the narratives from both people who were sighted and visually impaired I would (apart from the email quoted within this chapter) only include the personal writing from people who were visually impaired. As Mike said, when you include people from outside the main narrative (visual impairment) it becomes something different, and for the moment I want the focus to be on visual impairment. Perhaps the next step is to draw sighted people into dialogue to start a new narrative.

Chapter Fourteen

Narrative Perspectives on Research

This chapter explores the experience of using narrative practices to explore the experience of living with a visual impairment and the impact the process has had on contributors. It includes a commentary entitled, "emancipatory research practices".

Journal August 2009
I seem to have moved from being a practitioner and researcher to becoming a social activist. No longer does it seem enough to think about the effect of visual impairment on identity claims or how to help individuals make sense of their lives. This seems more about political campaigning, about developing a collective voice that is listened to. Kennedy's inaugural speech comes into mind:

> "Now the trumpet summons us again – not as a call to bear arms, though arms we need – not as a call to battle, though embattled we are – but a call to bear the burden of a long twilight struggle, year in and year out, 'rejoicing in hope, patient in tribulation' a struggle against the common enemies of man: tyranny, poverty, disease and war itself" (Kennedy 1961).

A twilight struggle it has become, a call to arms for visually impaired people to have their say. Perhaps the dissertation needs to be written into a book which will be available to wider audiences?

This is the final chapter of the book, yet strangely it feels like a beginning and the start of something rather than an end. The narratives remain "messy' (Marcus 1994) (cited by Speedy 2007), where as Speedy points out there "is a move away from neatly connected and completed work that has had its inconsistencies and contradictions and non-commensurate stories 'smoothed away'" (Speedy 2007:20).

We have told our stories, laughed a lot, cried a lot and struggled with literature and dominant discourses that surround blindness. We have challenged the use of text based academic practices, but still produced a text. We have tried to open up a space that will encourage other visually impaired people to have a voice, and tried to start a conversation and dialogue with sighted people in ways that do not overshadow the thoughts and experiences of those who are visually impaired.

For those of you who like a neat "happy ever after" ending I am sorry, but we are really not ready to end yet! There is no conclusion, only our thoughts as we consider the research process, and our lives linked by visual impairment. This chapter hopefully gives you a glimpse of the starting point of the next conversations. These "next" conversations may not be between the contributors, but will hopefully be taken up by others, and there will be meaningful dialogue between those who are sighted and those who are visually impaired.

"But are you not going to analyse these narratives?" I hear you ask, and the answer is perhaps "yes" and "no". Yes, in that we have all reflected on what we have said, and perhaps drawn out themes that were important to us, and no, in that we consider that the narratives are the analysis of the data which has been conversational and a co-construction of our lived experience. The narratives do not point to a fundamental "truth" which was there prior to our conversations, but because of who we are, and how we have talked together the conversations have constructed possibilities about how we are now and as we share these stories with you, and they are published they change and we become different. As Salmon points out:

> "All narratives are, in a fundamental sense, co-constructed. The audience, whether physically present or not, exerts a crucial influence on what can and cannot be said, how things should be expressed, what can be taken for granted, what needs explaining and so on. We now recognize that the personal account, in research interviews which has traditionally been seen as the expression of a single subjectivity, is in fact always a co-construction" (Salmon (forthcoming); Riessman 2008: quoting).

I asked all the contributors if there was anything else they would like to say about their experiences or the research and writing processes to readers of the book:

Sarah emails me:

Hello Sue,
Thank you for sending the chapters of the book written so far. I felt so emotional reading it. Being part of something, standing alongside other participants and reading their words alongside my own has been amazing. Life, as I've said to you before, has changed so much since I met you at the counselling service at Bristol. Then I felt so lost and lonely, and was in so much pain. Now I feel very differently, far more connected to others and I have my life back. Not the same

life, but a different one, and in some ways it is better because instead of thinking about me, me, me all the time I am thinking about other people. I talked to one elderly lady the other day about the angels I used to see (the Charles Bonnet Syndrome) and she then told me all about her hallucinations and how she was really frightened by them.

I still find living with this wretched eye condition frustrating, and often other people's attitudes are appalling, but there are some people out there who are actually interested and the more I talk about what has happened to me the more I find them.

I look forward to seeing the book in its final form!

Email from Will:

Hi Sue,
What an amazing journey we have come on. It seems such a long time since we first met over in Norway for the narrative therapy conference, and I only attended your workshop because you were visually impaired and I thought a bit of solidarity was needed!

I have learnt so much about myself and my relationship with visual impairment. I guess most of the time normally I put it right to the back of my mind and just fit in with all the sighted folks around me. I have started up a face book account where several of us who are visually impaired share our thoughts feelings and writing and give each other a bit of moral support. I hope that we will not lose touch now the book is on its way?

I talk with Annie:

Annie: Having you listen to me,
take me seriously,
ask me my opinions….
You don't know how much that means….
or perhaps you do?

Sue: Listening is something that doesn't always happen..
does it?

Annie: No.
People make judgements all the time.
It's quite strange
When you listen to me,
when I hear myself speaking,
it's like I can then move forward a bit more.
Reading other people's stories has been amazing,
some of them are the same as my experiences
some of them are different..
We are not all the same are we?

But there is always a sense of being in it together.

It's like we are speaking together about these things,
and this changes how we feel about them.
I still think how we are treated at the hospitals..
It is really shocking.
Seeing my experience written down I felt really,
really angry.
Before I just felt sad,
but seeing it written made me really mad.
And I am so glad to feel angry...

How can we get these kind of things changed do you think?

Sue: I guess we have to keep highlighting..
keep saying this is not right for people...

I have sent a copy of what you sent me to my MP
I think that he ought to lobby the government
to do something.
There are so many people, who have such
negative attitudes,
and it is not just the hospitals..
I went to the local "blind club" the other week..
It was awful.....
Well the people going to the club were ok,
they just had to do as they were told,
but the people running it...
it reminded me of something Tony said;
"would you like a nice cup of tea dear?"
So patronising it made me seethe...
Sorry Sue I'm going off on one!..

Sue: It sounds really important..
this anger...
fighting for justice.

Annie: Yes, I see this book as a call to arms
A call to others to join the campaign,
without being able to talk to you,
to read other people's stories has been
So important.

Email from Stephen

Hi Sue,
Yes I am still happy for you to include my emails in the book.
Reading what has been written has been a real eye opener (well
perhaps not literally because I'm blind). I still find it really difficult to
cope with blindness it is as if part of me has been taken away. I do
feel more able to talk about it now though. I don't seem to be

waiting on the hospital all the time, I am getting on best I can and living my life. I have started to learn long cane which is a very big thing, before I couldn't stand the thought of using a white cane, I just felt very embarrassed by the whole thing.

Email from Patrick

Hello Sue,
I was probably your most reluctant participant! To start with I was really ambivalent about sharing my experiences with people who were sighted. How could they ever understand? I thought, and did I really want them to? There was something for me about real fear that the life I thought I was so successful at would turn out to be negative, that I would crumble and fall to pieces.

It hasn't been like that at all though, I feel much less fearful, sharing my experiences and having them validated by others has meant I feel stronger and I don't avoid those losing sight now, I just realise that they are going through a stage of their journey, one which having someone positive like me around helps them with.

Being given permission to write about my feelings of rage and sadness has been very liberating. If I dwell on them too much then it feels quite overwhelming but I am so glad to have been involved in your project.

What are we going to do next?

Email from Dennis:

Hi Sue,

Have been thinking about your book and would like to include this:

Tragic or Heroic?
I first met Sue Dale at a BACP diversity conference about 6 years ago. It was the above titled description of how the general public often view visually impaired people that we quickly realised was of mutual interest. We both recognised that this was a perception that needed to be discussed, explored and indeed challenged!

I have macular degeneration and have been visually impaired for more than 30 years. The vast majority of blind and partially sighed people acquire sight problems during their life and go through a considerably difficult period of loss. Suffering such a keen sense of loss and experiencing grief because of it is a traumatic event. It is not made easier by the stoic "stiff upper lip" culture of the British when facing adversity.

Sue and I have since spent many hours discussing in depth our own feelings and experiences and how we have met and continue to meet the challenges of living in the world of the sighted.

Feeling low and even sorry for oneself attracts sympathy from others but also carries the threat of patronisation. Feelings of low self esteem and loss of independence will only exacerbate the problems. However, taking it "on the chin" and "getting on with it" leads to praise and even admiration. However I do feel that, even in the latter circumstances, the threat of patronisation still looms.

In the past I have been described as inspirational and amazing so I'm a little puzzled about experiencing feelings of some discomfort when I hear such praise.

I'm not heroic, or tragic; I don't want to be seen as inspirational either. I just want to be normal, whatever that means, to run with the pack, and be accepted and included as one of the crowd. If I'm not I might become isolated! When I'm referred to as a "visually impaired person" it sets me aside. As a "person who is visually impaired" I feel more included.

Giving people the opportunity to tell their story in a safe and confidential setting, to openly express thoughts and feelings, can be a considerably enabling event.

Emancipatory Research Practices

Most of the research connected with visual impairment comes, as I stated earlier, from medical models of understanding with emphasis on treatment and rehabilitation and even the small (but growing) research into the social and emotional welfare of people who are blind and partially sighted comes from "expert" understandings of what blindness and partial sight may mean (Burmedi et al. 2002; Stephens 2007). Although all of this research is valuable, and gives an understanding of the overall picture, it often renders those to whom the research is about, people such as myself, invisible and without a voice.

We (the visually impaired) I understand, are more likely to "show a decline in mental health, especially the occurrence of depression" (O'Neill and Harnindranath 2006:162; Burmedi et al. 2002:47; Stephens 2007:35; Horowitz and Reinhardt 2005:181-197; Horowitz, Reinhardt, and Kennedy 2005:625; Hinds et al. 2003:1391; Rovener 2001:1097-1100; De-Leo et al. 1999:341) and anxiety, and loneliness (Stephens 2007) than "normal" populations. We become less socially active (Burmedi et al. 2002). Our psychosocial activities are disrupted when we have to learn new skills and adjust to changing social relations (Stephens 2007). We are more likely to remain single and not working (Stephens 2007;

Nicholls 2004; Dale 2008), we may not feel "safe to carry out activities outside the home environment" (Girdhar et al. 2002 cited by Stephens 2007:14).

Whilst these studies do give us an overview, and highlight the need for more emphasis to be placed on the emotional needs of people who have lost sight, and this is a new good initiative, as in the past blindness was only considered in terms of the medical cause of not seeing (Kinash 2005) but, when I start to use the word "we" in respect to these words; "depression", "anxiety", "isolation", rather than "they" (the blind or partially sighted) I start to feel uncomfortable. Where does my personal experience fit into this maze? Where do the other individuals I have had the privilege of talking to fit? There is no room for individuality, or detail within these kind of quantitative figures, and nothing from the people affected by the issues directly. They may have filled in questionnaires, or even attended focus groups, or interviews, but their voice seems lost in all of this.

It is interesting to note that a study carried out in 1999 by Duckett and Pratt that called for visual impairment research, where there was, "greater inclusion of visually impaired people in such research and participatory, empowering and emancipatory research was a priority for them" (cited by:Duckett and Pratt 2007:7) but that when the recommendations of the study were looked at again in 2007 it was noted, "we risk plagiarizing ourselves – after updating our review of the research literature we were only able to find one example of such work (except for our own journal article published in 2001" (Duckett and Pratt 2007:7).

If indeed we, as visually impaired people, are isolated depressed and anxious, then keeping us "voiceless" as well as "sight-less" would seem a good way of keeping us that way! Recently I was asked to take part in a quantitative study looking at the work patterns of visually impaired adults, and I was delighted to have been asked, but increasingly frustrated by a questionnaire that was only interested in my views within very firm boundaries of "yes" and "no". I was able to say "I have had periods of employment lasting more than 2 years", but I was unable to voice what it is like trying to find and maintain work if you cannot "drive" and need longer to read and assimilate information. I guess all of the 500 or so people within the sample could have given much fuller richer answers. Will this research be portrayed as the "truth" about the work patterns of people who are blind and partially sighted, or as one of the "many possibilities that exist" I wonder?

Etherington comments that "life is both temporal and storied" (Etherington 2000:297). My experience of the world is both shaped by my gender, my age, my health, my sensory perceptions, all physical individual factors but, also I consider by social factors, the society that I live in, the relationships I have with other people, and the stories I tell (both to others and to myself) to make sense of all of these things. If our research only gives insight into the "temporal" and medical, but not the "storied" experiential part of life, then surely this is not a true representation of people's lived experience.

As Clandinin and Connelly state, "for us, life – as we come to it and as it comes to others – is filled with narrative fragments, enacted in storied moments of time and space, and reflected upon and understood in terms of narrative unities and discontinuities' (Clandinin and Connelly 2000:17). If we view the world as constructed through the relationships and the stories we tell of our lives (White and Epston 1990) then we need to find ways of constructing our identities that do not limit us to being a statistic on the page, or being "the blind" or "the visually impaired", a homogenous group, lacking the individual "storied" experience.

Speedy speaks of her work as "an invitation into conversation" (Speedy 2007:xiv) and the aim of this book is indeed conversation, conversations with each other about the stories of our lives, and conversations with people who may not have a personal experience of living with a visual impairment, or if they have, then their experience will again be unique and valued.

The word emancipatory means "release from control or restraint" or "freed from social convention" (Oxford English Dictionary). So, for research with a group who are silenced to be emancipatory, it needs to free the people who are being researched to have a voice other than what social convention and the researcher dictates. French and Swain have a bolder view of emancipatory research and write:

> "In terms of emancipatory intentions, a key question is: does research support disabled people in their struggle against oppression and the removal of barriers to equal opportunities and a full participatory democracy for all?" (French and Swain 2000:51)

Perhaps all researchers can ever do is aspire to these ideals, but, if we can even in a small way open up spaces for people who are affected by the issues (people such as myself, and the contributors in this book) to be heard within, or alongside the expert opinion and statistics, then this may enable us to have choices, and room to explore our relationship with these opinions and statistics, and freedom to decide what we might want to do, or not do in response, or even for us to explore how we have managed not to be isolated, anxious or depressed, and how we live fulfilling lives. Speedy speaks of how invitation to inhabit these spaces allows us to move towards "constructing our identities not as 'nouns' thus fixed, albeit open to change, but as 'verbs' and as discursive processes may lead us into more creative (and messier) research conversations" (Speedy 2007:42).

Using the stories people tell of their lives within a research conversation (often called narrative practices) is one way of opening up these spaces, because it gives people affected by the issues a voice, which often cuts across the grain of the "expert" or academic voices and questions taken for granted practices. Stories invite conversation and through conversation further stories emerge (White 2000) and the single voices become veritable choirs and that indeed does invite a "full participatory democracy for all".

Narrative practices have become one of the tools used by social scientists to explore not the generalities but the "particularities of certain lives and social worlds" (Speedy 2007:40). Narrative studies such as Hooks (1994); Brown, Gollop et al. (1997); Behan (1999); Etherington (2000); Langellier (2001); Luttrell (2002); Riessman (2006); Etherington (2008), enable the voices of people who traditionally have not been heard, people in the margins of society (Hooks 1994) to speak.

It is in the act of telling personal narratives we write or tell ourselves into being; as Josselson and Lieblich state, "we are the stories we tell" (Josselson, Lieblich, and McAdams 2003:3). This implies that it is possible in the process of re-writing to change how we describe our lives. As a therapist influenced by narrative practices I have noticed that people often do come as White states, "with thin problem saturated stories of their lives" (White 1995:16), and that by exploring alternative stories of their lives the descriptions they have of themselves become "rich and thick" and full of hope rather than despair.

The stories we tell within this study will not be the whole of what we are however. How could any of us sum up our complicated lives within a few minutes conversation or a few emails. We tell stories about our self differently according to the audience that listens, and as soon as the words leave us and are received by another our experience changes.

I do not anticipate that any of us will have the same descriptions of our lives now at the end of this process. Life has moved on for us. We become immersed in the mundane ordinary life experiences. The conversations we had about the research, the editing, the choosing, the further conversations all have an effect on how we would describe our lives (even the descriptions of being blind or partially sighted).

There is something about the "telling" or writing which constructs a different sense of self however. At the beginning of this book I referred to Kleege (1999) who opens her book with the sentence, "writing this book made me blind", and how through the writing she created and described herself, as "blind". This was a defiant positive description (Kleege 2006; Mintz 2007) which came about only through the process of the life story being told. Mintz comments that Kleege's writing "redefines the meaning of blindness not so much by attempting to establish an equivalency between vision and blindness but, rather by 'disabling' sightedness itself" (Mintz 2007:72). To many who are sighted this will seem a very uncomfortable process, but it is only by challenging the taken for granted assumptions that to be sighted is normal that we can start thinking about the experience of visual impairment from a visually impaired perspective. Frank talks about the desire in common culture for restitution narratives and comments that "contemporary culture treats health as the normal condition that people ought to have restored.",(Frank 1995:77) so living with a permanent visual impairment where sight is not restored, and in some cases is not even desired, does not conform to the societal norm. This means that stories which do not have the plot of "searching for a cure" or "overcoming adversity" remain on the margins. We are supposed to "fight" illness or in the case of visual impairment loss of sight, but as Martin comments about her own illness "I remember being aware that the conventional 'wisdom' about serious illness was that one is supposed to fight. I was not at all sure how I might go about this supposed fight, with its implications of winning and losing" (Martin 2011:104). These war like metaphors may help some individuals, but for many pose an additional hurdle over which they are expected to identify their lives. Hopefully by constructing these narratives in ways which avoid these war filled metaphors there has been opportunity for other stories to emerge which are more helpful in defining what it means to us to be visually impaired.

One of the aspects of this telling of stories that has had a significant influence on how we define our lives now, and indeed the narratives you read in this book, is the concept that when an individual tells a story of their lives which is witnessed by another who allows what they have heard to resonate with their own life experiences, there is a change in how both the story teller and the witness then identify themselves. If how we describe our lives is influenced by social processes then the telling of stories about our lives, and the witnessing of those stories, becomes a dynamic process resulting in changes to all those involved. The life stories contained in a book such as this become more than just evidence of an experience that happened at some time in the past, but become part of the process of redefining where we are now. Witnessing in this way has parallels with the narrative practices of "definitional ceremony"

Definitional Ceremony and Outsider Witness Practices

Barbara Myerhoff (Myerhoff 1982, 1986) who coined the phrase "definitional ceremony" was an anthropologist who worked with an ageing Jewish community in Los Angeles. She discovered that the way in which they kept their fragmenting community together was to tell stories of their lives and culture in front of witnesses, and then for the witnesses to re-tell the stories with their own experiences, and this re-defined their sense of belonging and strengthened their fragile community. She called this process "definitional ceremony". The definitional ceremonies,

> "contrived to allow people to reiterate their collective and personal identities, to arouse great emotion and energy which was then redirected toward some commonalities, some deep symbols, and stable shared norms" (Myerhoff 1979:185),

and the concept has been taken up within the narrative therapy movement [and also by narrative researchers (Speedy 2007)] to enable previously marginalised people to re-define their lives in ways that are "richer and thicker" and build a sense of community. (White 2001).

Within the therapeutic and research uses of definitional ceremony this usually means that the person at the centre of the process (the client or the research participant) is asked to tell their story (facilitated by an interviewer) to a group of witnesses, these could be family members, or people who have had similar life experiences often called "outsider witnesses" (Fox, Tench, and Marie 2003). After the telling the person at the centre of the process moves to the position of the audience and the witnesses are interviewed about what they have heard in terms of; identifying the expression which struck a chord that the person's story evoked; what these expressions suggested about the person's purposes, values, hopes, dreams and commitments; what personal aspects of the witnesses own life resonated with the person's story. Also whether the stories have impacted on the witnesses and taken them to a place they would not otherwise have experienced (White 2000). The person at the centre of the process would then re-tell their story in light of these comments, and often the story would have evolved to include feelings of linking lives around common themes and be experienced as re-defining in positive ways (Behan 1999).

It would seem as we tell our stories of living with a visual impairment, other people, informally, resonate in the way of the definitional ceremony witnesses, and tell their own stories and how they resonate with ours, and this helps us to re-define who we are and the communities to which we belong. Certainly as I have read, transcribed and edited the stories from all of the contributors I have resonated with many aspects of their stories, and this has changed my perception of who I am. I am more able to speak of belonging to a group of people who are visually impaired, but not totally blind. We have collaborated to produce a collective narrative that shows the process of research, and also challenges sighted stereotypical attitudes about blindness and visual impairment.

Messy Texts

Creating collaboratively written narratives does pose problems for the researcher however, as Speedy states they are messy (Speedy 2005:42) and ethically challenging. It is not sufficient to ensure the participants sign a paper confirming they have given "informed consent" to their words being used. As the narrative of the research process unfolds, the "informed" bit changes with each word added. How can you at the beginning give "informed consent" to such a dynamic process where you do not know what the end result will be unless you constantly remain vigilant, and as the researcher, always hold the participants in mind. As Etherington states "I have tried to imagine all of them reading what I am writing, what they might think, feel, want or not want, while at the same time being true to myself" (Etherington 2000:298).

It interests me that in traditional research paradigms ethical research has often meant that the identity of the participants is protected at all costs, and indeed this means that the participants can say what they want to without anyone being able to identify them. I wonder however, alongside all the benefits this may have, how this works for people who feel that they want a voice, and if anonymity is another way they feel that they are being silenced and rendered invisible. Atkinson and Williams include names and even photographs of participants within an anthology of prose, poetry and art by people with learning difficulties (Atkinson and Williams 1990), and I notice how this inclusion draws me into relationship with specific individuals and their unique lived experience rather than thinking of them as "people with learning disabilities".

Talking with contributors to this book, it became clear that they wanted some level of privacy and for them to be in control of how that happened. This has meant that they have chosen whether or not to use their real names or pseudonyms, whether they want contact with the other participants, or within any presentations of the study, what they want to say to audiences and what these decisions might mean for them, or for their families. It is surely part of the emancipatory process that people are given autonomy to choose to be involved or not, and to the level that suits them.

Another ethical dilemma particular to this project is that the visual impaired community is a small one, and I have known many of the contributors in a number of different roles, and they have all known me as a "counsellor" whether that be as a colleague, supervisor, client, or from my writing. Some of them have also known each other in different roles, and I was conscious that the research process and writing of the book might affect these. Josselson says, "Do you really feel like interfering in his or her life? Will you be able to live with the consequences of this encounter or intervention? Is it justified from the interviewee's own perspective?" (Josselson 1996:9 cited by Etherington 2000:265). All very relevant comments, and the only way of countering them was to talk to the people concerned, and be as transparent as possible about the process.

Again, sharing information, being transparent, seems more libratory than "taking responsibility" for all the decisions about the project. I am aware however that I do stand in a different position to the others within this book in that I am acting as editor, and have chosen which contributions to include and where they are placed, but hopefully I making these decisions in a collaborative rather than autocratic way!

Emancipation however is not just about "having a voice", but as the psalmist says, it is also about "breaking the chains" (psalm 2:3) or to put it another way; actions speak louder than words.

Having a voice is indeed very important and sharing stories amongst ourselves will change how we view the world. However, if no-one outside listens to our voices, then it would leave public and professional opinion untouched. Clinicians will still treat people as "a pair of eyes" and the public would still see us as "pitiful". A book such as this will have a narrow audience, but hopefully it will prove a starting point and encourage others to speak out. I have learnt from presenting the stories of our experiences to diverse audiences, that despite societal prejudice, many people are receptive and do say; "I never really thought about visual impairment in that way", some ophthalmologists and other health professionals are (despite overcrowded clinics) trying to treat people as more than just "eyes". Dennis had a conversation with one recently who said, "I try and treat everyone as if he or she were my relative, with that level of respect", but it feels sometimes that there is a long way to go.

Andy emails:

Hi Sue,
Good to hear from you again. I was amazed by the chapters of the book you sent.

It seems a long time ago that we had our first conversations, reading what I said then seems really strange. I was so very angry. I guess that I am still angry about some things; like the attitudes of the hospital and other specialists who I think should know better. I think I've got a bit more tolerant of the general public – well with a white cane they mostly stay out of my way and that's fine! Or is it?

I have started doing an Open University course on psychology because as I've read all the stuff we have written together it has really interested me. The way people think, and how that affects what they do and how they get on in life seems really important. I've also got divorced which although painful was the right thing for both of us. The relationship was going wrong way before I lost my sight, that I think was the final straw and I could never be the person she wanted me to be.

Being involved with these various projects with you has meant getting my self-esteem and confidence back. That has partly been due to my contact with you, and you saying that what I had to say was worth something, but it's also about the other people involved and feeling part of something rather than an outsider isolated by blindness. I have started meeting up with Patrick and Caroline (who also have contributed to this book) and we are thinking about writing something together and that feels really exciting.

Beth sends a poem:

Alone and isolated I stood
Unsure, unwelcome, unwanted.
My non-sight a barrier to all.

Who I was grew smaller
Diminished, disparaged, denied
until I thought nothing, was worth nothing
a silent victim to be pitied.
A victim who did not even fight for sight.

Other people have now joined me,
vibrant, strident, with non-sighted vision,

I sing in a choir of blind voices,
A community formed with a mission.

Mo writes to me:

Dear Sue,
I never ever thought that I would be a contributor in a book, I never
thought that I had anything useful to say. I have so enjoyed reading
what others have written, and feel part of something very special.

Thank you for making an old woman feel that she is worth
something.

p.s. I do hope that all doctors at eye hospitals read this and start
treating people differently.

All of us have said that we feel in a very different place from
when we started the project. The sharing of our lives linked by a
common theme has enabled us to think differently about how we
relate to our visual impairment, and how we have relationships with
others, both sighted, and visually impaired.

We have tried to make sense of our lives as visually impaired
people, lived as they are within societal perceptions of what
blindness and sight loss mean, and recognise as Holstein and
Gubrium point out that "social pressure, as we are coming to realize
have the power of a glacier" (Holstein and Gubrium 2000:8).
Glaciers can change the shape of the landscape dramatically, so
sighted perceptions have affected our sense of self and identity. At
the front of glaciers however are small mountain streams, and we
hope that this small stream of conversation will be joined by other
conversations and this will lead one day to the formation of a
mighty river which will also have the power to apply social pressure
for change.

We have thought about culture and identity and examined how
being visually impaired impacts on our sense of self. We have
worked our way through themes; relating to our relationship with
the sighted world, the commonly held assumptions about blindness,
our personal relationships with sighted others, about feelings of
being isolated and marginalised, our feelings about not being
sighted; and yet not being completely blind, our experiences of
growing up, education, social injustice and much more. We have
engaged with literature relating to narrative research methodologies,
social construction theories, emancipatory research practices, visual
impairment research, disability studies, cultural studies, and
narrative therapy.

We have used our conversations to construct identities both individually, and as a group, and through the group felt empowered and enabled to have a voice. We have "performed" excerpts of these conversations within a narrative in order to enable us to engage in a "performative struggle over meanings" (Riessman 2008:106) and to engage with you in a dialogue about sight and blindness, and enable you to glimpse the lived experience people who are visually impaired. As Hull says,

> "we understand that blindness is not only something that happens to your eyes but is a world creating condition. Sight is also a world creating condition but sighted people do not usually realise this" (Hull 1999:70).

At an international therapy conference the late Michael White was asked about the goals of narrative therapy and he said "it is quite simple. To turn thin problem saturated stories into thick rich narratives of people's lives" (White 2007 verbal quotation at conference). Although this book is not "narrative therapy", in that it was entered into as a co-researched project to explore our experience of visual impairment, the goals have been similar, and we have indeed moved from thin stories of what visual impairment meant to us, to thick rich descriptions and this has for all of us proved therapeutic.

When I started researching with others their experiences of living with a visual impairment I identified myself as a counsellor and researcher. I have finished by writing a book and somewhat to my own surprise now define myself as a "social activist"! Because, although I was seeking to understand more about how a visual impairment affected identity, what perhaps has become more important, is the question of how we as a minority group linked by visual impairment can overcome and challenge the societal prejudice and privilege of sight, and the aesthetic, in order to be able to participate fully, and become integral respected parts of our communities.

EPILOGUE

THE RE-GRILLING OF MR. B

Grilling:
    1. is a form of cooking that involves direct heat. Devices that grill are called "grills"
    2. an act or process of interrogating a person in an intimidating and persistent manner
(Encarta Dictionary English UK)

Journal 24th November 2007

I visited May and Peter today. I wanted to talk to them about what I had written about the "grilling of Mr. B".

"Of course you can use it...if you think that it will be of interest to anyone apart from us" said May. "We did enjoy it. Not often we get to play at our age…….. It helped us though, and that what makes all the difference" said Peter.

As I trundle home on the train and recall their words, I have the distinct feeling that they were laughing at me for taking myself so seriously. I feel a sense of being very privileged to have listened to their stories from so many decades, I have learnt so much from my work with them, and I feel sad too because this is an ending. Although I am sure that if I telephoned and asked if I could visit again they would say yes, I know that they do not need me in my role as therapist any more, and I guess that I will not see them again.

Journal 8th Jan 2008

I received a postcard from Peter and May today and on the front was a poem by Spike Milligan:

"A thousand hairy savages
Sitting down to lunch
Gobble, gobble, glup, glup
Munch, munch, munch"
(with a cartoon drawing of the savages)

.

On the back Peter and May had written:

"This is us and your readers eating Mr. B for lunch. Thank you. You helped us so much (and your interrogation techniques were brilliant) it was so good to talk about it with you. I hope it helps others to vanquish their Mr. B's.
With regards,
Peter and May"

Journal September 21st 2010
I received a letter from May and Peter's daughter today:

Dear Sue,
Dad asked me to write to you as he thought that you would want to know the news.

Mum died peacefully in her sleep two weeks ago, although I miss her very much she was 88 and had a good life.

I came across the article you had written about the "Grilling of Mr. B" amongst her things. Both she and dad have often talked about it, and even played the audio version to various family members. There was something about that conversation that was deeply significant to their lives together. Certainly over the last couple of years both Mum and Dad have seemed very at peace with the world.

It is even more poignant now because at the age of 62 I have now also been diagnosed with macular degeneration, and have already lost significant sight. I keep a copy of the Mr. B script above my desk to remind me that I can survive this and that blindness can be overcome. Every time I read it I feel connected to Mum and that is a gift too precious for words.

Dad is living with us now as he found the house to difficult to manage alone. He sends his regards though and a request for a copy of the book when it's out.

Yours sincerely
Maureen

BIBLIOGRAPHY

Atkinson, D, and F Williams, eds. 1990. *Know me as I am: an anthology of prose, poetry and art by people with learning difficulties*. London: Hodder and Stoughton.

Atkinson, R. 2007. Do I want my sight back? . *The Guardian July 17th 2007*.

Barkham, M, J Mellor-Clark, J Connell, and J Cahill. 2006. A core approach to practice-based evidence: a brief history of the origins and applications of the CORE-OM and CORE System. *Counselling and Psychotherapy Research,* 6 (1):3-15.

Barnes, C, and G Mercer. 2003. *Disability, Key Concepts*. Cambridge: Polity Press.

Barnes, C, G Mercer, and T Shakespeare. 1999. *Exploring disability: A sociological introduction*. Cambridge: Polity Press.

Batra, M, M Bartels, and H Wormstall. 2009. Therapeutic options in Charles Bonnet Syndrome. *Acta psychiatrica Scandinavica* 96 (2):129-33.

Behan, C. 1999. Linking lives around shared themes: narrative group therapy with gay men. *Gecko: A journal of deconstruction and narrative ideas in therapeutic practice* vol.2.

Bingham, J Clifton 1927. Just a song at twilight. In *The Community Song Book 3rd edition*, edited by S. Campbell. London: Lovello.

Bolt, D. 2005. Caught in the chasm: literary representation and suicide among people with impaired vision. *The British journal of visual impairment* 23 (3):117-121.

Brockmeier, J, and D Carbaugh, eds. 2001. *Narrative and Identity*. Edited by J. Brockmeier and D. Carbaugh, *Narrative and Identity*. Amsterdam: John Benjamins Publishing Company.

Brown, GW, CJ Gollop, MG Goodson, P Green-Powell, A Hambrick, LA Kingham, J Moody, C Obbo, EA Peterson, DD Turner, KM Vaz, J Walcott-McQuigg, and RT White. 1997. *Oral narrative research with black women*. Edited by K. M. Vaz. London: Sage Publications.

Burmedi, D, S Becker, V Heyl, H Wahl, and I Himmelsbach. 2002. Emotional and social consequences of age-related low vision; a narrative review. *Visual Impairment Research* 4 (1):47-71.

Butler, S. 2007. Out of sight out of mind? *in focus* Spring 2007:24-33.

Campbell, J, and M Oliver. 1996. *Disability Politics: Understanding our past, changing our future*. London: Routledge.

Ching, L. 1980. *One of the lucky ones*. Kowloon, Hong Kong: Ocean Printing Co. Ltd.

Clandinin, DJ, and FM Connelly. 2000. *Narrative inquiry*. San Fransisco: Jossey-Bass.

Cloke, P, P Cooke, J Cursons, P Milbourne, and R Widdowfield. 2000. Ethics, Reflexivity and Research: Encounters with homeless people. *Ethics, Place and Environment* 3 (2):133-154.

Dale, S. 2006. Knitting in the dark: narratives about the experience of sight loss: Unpublished Doctoral assignment University of Bristol.

—. 2006. Knitting in the Dark: Two personal accounts: RNIB Unpublished audio recordings used for training purposes.

—. 2008. The Grilling of Mr B: Using the narrative therapy practice of 'externalising' conversations to co-research the experience of blindness: Bristol University.

—. 2008. Report on the RNIB Bristol Counselling project 2005-2008. London: RNIB.

—. 2008a. Knitting in the dark: narratives about the experience of sight loss in a counselling setting. *British Journal of Visual Impairment* September 2008.

—. 2008b. Casting Off: using narrative practices to co-research experiences of sight loss and visual impairment. *TSI-Theory in Action* 1 (2).

—. 2008c. *Different Horizons: Counselling People who are blind and partially sighted*. London: RNIB Publications.

—. 2009. EdD thesis: Songs at twilight:: A narrative exploration of the experience of living with a visual impairment, and the effect this has on identity claims., Graduate School of Education University of Bristol, Bristol.

—. 2009. The Grilling of Mr B: Using the narrative therapy practice of 'externalising' conversations to co-research the experience of blindness. *Therapy Today September 2009* 20 (7).

—. 2009. The Grilling of Mr. B. *Therapy Today September 2009* 20 (7):24-27.

—. 2010. *Where angels fear to tread: having conversations about suicide in a counselling context*. Newcastle upon Tyne: Cambridge Scholars Publishing.

Davies, B, S Gannon, S Laws, C Rocco, H Taguchi, and H McCann. 2001. Becoming Schoolgirls: the ambivalent process of subjectification. *Gender and Education* 13 (2) 167-182.

Davies, R. 2007. Substance Misuse Counselling workforce shortages: Welsh Assembly Government.

De-Leo, D., P Hickey, G Meneghel, and C Cantor. 1999. Blindness, fear of sight loss and suicide. *Psychosomatics* July-August 1999, 40 (4):339-344.

Douglas, G, S Pavey, B Clements, and C Concoran. 2009. Network 1000: Visually impaired people's access to employment: Visual Impairment Centre for Teaching and Research (VICTAR): University of Birmingham.

Douglas, G, S Pavey, and C Corcoran. 2008. Access to information services and support for people with visual impairment. In *Network 1000*, edited by VICTAR. Birmingham: Vision 2020 UK and University of Birmingham.

Duckett, P, and R Pratt. 2007. The emancipation of visually impaired people in social science research practice. *British Journal of Visual Impairment* 25 (5).

Ellis, C. 1999. Heartful Autoethnography. *Qualitative Health Research* Vol. 9 (5):669-683.

Ellis, C , and MG Flaherty. 1992. *Investigating subjectivity: research on lived experience*. London: Sage publications.

Ellis, C, and A Bochner. 1992. Telling and performing personal stories. In *Investigating subjectivity*, edited by C. Ellis and A. Bochner. London: sage publications.

—. 2000. Auto ethnography, personal narrative reflexivity: researcher as subject. In *Handbook of qualitative research*, edited by N. K. Denzin and Y. Lincoln. London: sage publications.

Eperjesis, F, and N Akbarali. 2009. Rehabilitation in Charles Bonnet Syndrome. *Optometry* 87 (3):149-152.

Etherington, K. 2000. *Narrative approaches to working with adult male survivors of child sexual abuse*. London: Jessica Kingsley publishers.

—. 2001. Research with ex-client's a celebration and extension of the therapeutic process. *British journal of guidance and counselling* 29 (1).

—. 2008. *Trauma, drug misuse and transforming identities: a life story approach*. London: Jessica Kingsley Publishers.

Ferguson, R.J., ed. 2001. *We know who we are: a history of the blind in challenging educational and socially constructed policies: A study in policy archaeology*. San Francisco: Caddo Gap.

Fitzgerald, R G, and C Murray Parkes. 1998. Blindness and loss of other sensory and cognitive functions. *BMJ* 316 (7138) (April 1998):1160-1163.

Fox, H, C Tench, and Marie. 2003. Outsider Witness practices and group supervision. *The International journal of narrative therapy and community work 2003* vol.4.

Frank, A W. 1995. *The wounded storyteller: body, illness, and ethics,* . Chicago, IL: University of Chicago Press.

Freedman, J, and G Combs. 1996. *Narrative Therapy: the social construction of preferred realities*. New York: W.W. Norton Company Inc.

Freeman, C. 2009. Middle Step: An evolving best practice model addressing the emotional needs of people with sight loss. Paper read at VINCE Conference 2009, at Birmingham.

French, S, and J Swain. 2000. Good intentions: reflecting on researching the lives and experiences of visually disabled people. *Annual Review of Critical Psychology* 2:35-54.

—. 2004. Whose tragedy? Towards a personal non-tragedy view of disability. In *Disabling barriers - enabling environments (2nd edition)*, edited by J. Swain, S. French, C. Barnes and Thomas. London: Sage.

French, S, J Swain, D Atkinson, and M Moore. 2006. *An oral history of the education of visually impaired children: telling stories for inclusive futures*. Lampeter: Edwin Mellen Press.

Girdhar, P, R Dandona, M.N Prasad, V Kovai, and L Dandona. 2002. Fear of blindness and perceptions about blind people: The Andhra Pradesh eye disease study. *Indian Journal of Ophthalmology* 50 (3):239-246.

Hahn, A. 2008. Macular Degeneration. London: http://www.adamhahn.co.uk/ accessed 23.11.2008.

Hinds, A, A Sinclair, J Park, A Suttie, H Patterson, and M Macdonald. 2003. Impact of interdisciplinary low vision service on the quality of life of low vision patients. *British Journal of Ophthalmology* 87:1391-1396.

Hodge, S., W. Barr, and P. Knox. 2010. Evaluation of Emotional Support and Counselling within an integrated low vision service: Health and Community Care Research Unit. University of Liverpool.

Hole, R.D. 2004. Narratives of identity: a poststructural analysis of three deaf women's life stories, University of British Columbia, University of British Columbia, Michigan.

Holstein, J, and J Gubrium. 2000. *The self we live by: narrative identity in a postmodern world*. Oxford, New York: Oxford University Press.

Hooks, B. 1994. *Teaching to transgress*. New York: Routledge.

Horowitz, A, J.P. Reinhardt, and G Kennedy. 2005. Major and subthreshold depression among older adults seeking vision rehabilitation services. *American Journal of Geriatric Psychiatry* 13:180-187.

Horowitz, A, and P Reinhardt. 2005. Adequacy of the mental health system in meeting the needs of adults who are visually impaired. *Aging and Mental Health* 94 (10):625-637.

Hull, J. 1990. *Touching the Rock*. New York: Vintage Books.

—. 1999. The material spirituality of blindness and money. In *Wrestling and resting*, edited by R. Harvey. London: CTBI.

Humphries, S, and P Gordon. 1992. *Out of sight: The experience of disability 1900-1950*. Plymouth: Northcote House Publishing.

Jones, L, and R Bunton. 2008. Wounded or warrior. In *Narrative Research in health and illness*, edited by B. Hurwitz, T. Greenhalgh and V. Skultans. Oxford: BMA - Blackwell publishing Ltd.

Josselson, R. 1996. Ethics and process. *The narrative study of lives* 4.

Josselson, R, A Lieblich, and D P McAdams. 2003. *Up close and personal: the teaching and learning of narrative research*. Washington: American psychological association.

Keller, H. 1912. *The story of my life: with her letters (1887-1901) and a supplementary account of her education*. London: Hodder and Stoughton.

—. 1933. *The world I live in*. London: Methuen and Co Ltd.

Kennedy, J.F. 1961. Inaugural address 20 January 1961. *Vital Speeches* no 227 (February 1961).

Kinash, S. 2005. *Seeing beyond blindness*. Edited by R. J. Ferguson, *Critical concerns in blindness*. Greenwich, Connecticut: Information Age Publishing.

Kleege, G. 1999. *Sight Unseen*. New Haven: Yale University Press.

—. 2006. *Blind Rage: letters to Helen Keller*. Washington D.C.: Gallaudet University Press.

Knighton, R. 2006. *Cockeyed: a memoir*. London: Atlantic Books.

———. 2007. Eyes Wide Shut. *Telegraph 27.10.2007*.

Krieger. 2005. Losing my vision. *Qualitative Inquiry* 11 (2):145-151.

Kuusisto, S. 1998. *planet of the blind*. London: Faber and Faber.

—. 2008. Of or pertaining to Neruda: http://kuusisto.typepad.com/planet_of_the_blind/2008/03/today-talk-of-t.html accessed 20.10.2008.

Langellier, K M. 2001. You're marked; breast cancer, tattoo, and the narrative performance of identity. In *Narrative and identity*, edited by J. Brockmeier and D. Carbaugh. Amsterdam: John Benjamins publishing company.

Luttrell, W. 2002. *Pregnant bodies fertile minds: gender, race and the schooling of pregnant teens*. London: Routledge.

Magee, B, and M Milligan. 1995. *On Blindness*. New York: Oxford Press.

Marcus, G. 1994. What comes just after 'post'?: The case of Ethnography. In *Handbook of Qualitative Research*, edited by N. Denzin and Y. Lincoln. Thousand Oaks: Sage.

Martin, V. 2011. *Developing a narrative approach to healthcare research*. Oxon: Radcliffe Publishing Ltd.

Maslow, A. H. 1968. *Towards a psychology of being*. New York: Van Nostrand Reinhold.

—. 1973. *The Farther Reaches of Human Nature*. Harmondsworth: Penguin.

McBride, S. 2005. Patients with severe sight loss; emotional support and counselling. *OT* September 23:36-37.

McLeod, J, and M Cooper. 2010. *Pluralistic Counselling and Psychotherapy*. London: Sage.

Meredith, P. 2008. A Half-Caste on the Half-Caste in the Cultural Politics of New Zealand: The University of Waikato External Publications. www.lianz.waikato.ac.nz accessed 5.11.08.

Mintz, S.B. 2007. *Unruly Bodies: Life writing by women with disabilities*. Chapel Hill: The University of North Carolina Press.

Monbeck, M. E. 1973. *The meaning of blindness: the attitudes toward blindness and blind people*. London: Indiana University Press.

Morgan, A. 2000. *What is narrative therapy? An easy to read introduction*. Adelaide: Dulwich Centre Publications.

Mower, O. 1962. Freud and theory of personality. *The Journal of Nervous and Mental Disease* 135 (4):378.

Myerhoff, B. 1979. *Number our days*. London. New York: Meridian published by Penguin group.

—. 1982. Life history among the elderly: Performance, visibility and remembering. In *A crack in the mirror: reflexive perspectives in anthropology*, edited by J. Ruby. Philadelphia: University of Pennsilvania.

—. 1986. Life not death in Venice: It's second life. In *The anthropology of experience*, edited by V. Turner and E. Bruner. Chicago: University of Illinois Press.

NFB. 2008. mission statement: http://www.nfb.org/nfb accessed 26.11.08.

Nicholls, T. 2004. RNIB Bristol Counselling Project Report: Department of Health Section 64 funded project September 2001-August 2004. London: RNIB.

Norcross, J.C., ed. 2005. *A primer on psychotherapy integration*. Edited by J. C. Norcross and G. M.R., *Handbook of psychotherapy integration*. New York: Oxford University.

Nyman, S.R. *The psychosocial impact of vision loss in older people: Generations Review 20 (2)* http://www.britishgerontology.org/10newsletter2 2010b [cited 20/10/10.

Nyman, S.R., M. A. Gosney, and C.R. Victor. 2010a. Emotional well-being in people with sight loss: Lessons from the grey literature. *British Journal of Visual Impairment* 28 (3):175-203.

O'Neill, M, and R Harnindranath. 2006. Theorising narratives of exile and belonging: The importance of biography and ethno-mimesis in 'understanding' asylum. *Qualitative Sociology Review* 2 (1).

Payne, M. 2000. *Narrative therapy*. London: Sage Publications.

Pelias, R. J. 1999. *Writing performance: poeticizing the researcher's body*. New York: Dump Eurospan.

Reissman, C, and J Speedy. 2006. Narrative inquiry in the psychotherapy professions: a critical review. In *The handbook of narrative inquiry*, edited by J. Clandinin. Thousand Oaks: Sage.

Richardson, L. 1990. *Writing strategies; reaching diverse audiences*. California: Sage publications.

—. 2000. Introduction- assessing alternative modes of qualitative and ethnographic research: how do we judge? Who judges? *Qualitative Inquiry* Vol 6 (2):251-252.

—. 2000. Writing: A method of Inquiry. In *Handbook of qualitative research*, edited by N. K. Denzien and Y. Lincoln. London: Sage Publications.

Richardson, L, V Taylor, and N (Editor) Whittier. 2000. *Feminist Frontiers*. New York: Mc Graw Hill Co Inc.

Richardson, L. 1992. The consequences of poetic representation: writing the other, re-writing the self. In *Investigating subjectivity: research on lived experience*, edited by C. a. F. Ellis, M. Newbury Park, CA: Sage.

—. 2003. Poetic representation of interviews In *Postmodern Interviewing*, edited by J. Gubrium and J. Holstein. London: Sage.

Riessman, C, K. 2008. *Narrative methods for the human sciences*. London: Sage.

RNIB. 2008. sight problems: http://www.rnib.org.uk/xpedio/groups/public/documents/publicw ebsite accessed 4.4.2008.

—. 2010. Rehabilitation services in the south west region: http://www.rnib.org.uk/aboutus/contactdetails/england/southwes t/Pages/swrehab.aspx accessed 03.06.2010.

Rogers, C. 1961. *On becoming a person*. London: Constable.

—. 1978. *On personal power*. London: Constable.

Rovener, B.W. 2001. Neuroticism predicts depression and disability in age-related macular degeneration. *American Geriatrics Society* 49 (8):1097-1100.

—. 2006. The Charles Bonnet Syndrome: a review of recent research. *Current opinion in ophthalmology* 17 (3):275-77.

Rowan, J. 1983. *The Reality Game: a guide to humanistic counselling and psychotherapy*. London: Routledge.

Runyan, M, and S Jenkins. 2001. *No finish line: My life as I see it*. New York: Berkley Books.

Salmon, P (forthcoming). Some thoughts on narrative research. In *Doing narrative research in the social sciences*, edited by M. Andrews, S. Squire and Tamboukou. London: Sage.

Schadlu, A.P, R Schadlu, and J.b Shepherd. 2009. Charles Bonnet Syndrome: a review. *Current opinion in ophthalmology* 20 (3):219-22.

Schinazi, V. R. 2007. Psychosocial implications of blindness and low-vision. *Centre for Advanced Spatial Analysis – University College London Royal London Society for the Blind (RLSB) UCL Working Papers Series* 1 (114).

Scott, R. A. 1969. *The making of blind men: a study of adult socialization*. London: Transaction Publishers.

Seeing-Sense. 2010. The role of ECLO http://seeing-sense.com accessed 28.10.10.

Smith, Linda Tuhiwa. 1999. *Decolonizing methodologies: research and indigenous peoples, oral history with marginalized groups*. London. New York: Zed books University of Otago Press.

Speedy. 2005. Writing as inquiry: some ideas and practices. *Counselling and psychotherapy research* 5 (1):65-73.

Speedy, J. 2004. Living a more peopled life: definitional ceremony as inquiry into therapy outcomes. *International Journal of Narrative Therapy and Community Work* 3:43-53.

—. 2005. Collective biography practices: collective writing with the unassuming geeks group. *Briish Journal of Psychotherapy Integration* 2 (2):29-38.

—. 2007. *Narrative Inquiry and Psychotherapy*. Houndsmill: Palgrave Macmillan.

Stephens, J. 2007. The Emotional well-being of blind and partially sighted people. London: Guide Dogs

Tedlock, D. 1983. *The spoken word and the work of interpretation*. Philadelphia: University of Pensylvania.

Thetford, C., J. Robinson, J. Mehta, P. Knox, and D. Wong. 2008. The changing needs of people with sight loss: Final report for Thomas Pocklington Trust Health and Community Care Research Unit, University of Liverpool.

Thurston, M. 2010. An inquiry into the emotional impact of sight loss and the counselling experience and needs of blind and partially sighted people. *Counselling and Psychotherapy Research,* 10 (1):3-12.

Tuttle, D, and N Tuttle. 2004. *Self Esteem and adjusting with blindness: the process of responding to life's demands*.

Vale, D. 2001. Improving Lives: Priorities in health and social care for blind and partially sighted people. London: RNIB.

White, C, ed. 1997. *Challenging disabling practices: talking about issues of disability*. Edited by D. C. Newsletter. Adelaide: Dulwich Publications.

White, M. 1985. Fear busting and monster training. *Dulwich Centre Review* (1985).

—. 1995. *Re-Authoring Lives*. Adelaide: Dulwich Centre.

—. 1999. Re-engaging with history: the absent but implicit. Paper read at The narrative therapy and community work conference, Adelaide, February 1999, at Adelaide.

—. 2000. Reflecting Teamwork as definitional ceremony revisited. In *Reflections on narrative practice: essays and interviews*, edited by M. White. Adelaide: Dulwich Centre Publications.

—. 2001. Narrative practice and the unpacking of identity conclusions. *Gecko: A journal of deconstruction and narrative practice* 2001 (1).

—. 2003. Definitional ceremony and outsider witness responses. In *narrative therapy and community work conference*. Adelaide: Dulwich Centre http://www.dulwichcentre.com.au accessed 30.5.07.

—. 2007. Working with trauma. Paper read at International Conference of Narrative Therapy and Community Work, at Norway.

White, M , and D Epston. 1990. *Narrative means to therapeutic ends*. New York: W.W. Norton and company.

Wileman, R.E. 1980. *Exercises in visual thinking*. New York: Hastings House.

INDEX OF CONTRIBUTORS

SUBJECT INDEX